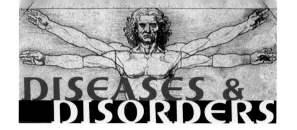

Flu

Titles in the Diseases and Disorders series include:

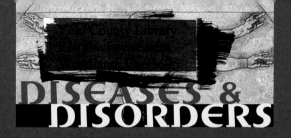

Flu

Barbara Sheen

LUCENT BOOKS

An imprint of Thomson Gale, a part of The Thomson Corporation

THOMSON

GALE

Detroit • New York • San Francisco • San Diego • New Haven, Conn.
Waterville, Maine • London • Munich

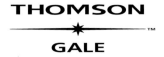

On cover: A colored chest X-ray shows lungs infected with the flu virus.

© 2007 Thomson Gale, a part of The Thomson Corporation.

Thomson and Star Logo are trademarks and Gale and Lucent Books are registered trademarks used herein under license.

For more information, contact
Lucent Books
27500 Drake Rd.
Farmington Hills, MI 48331-3535
Or you can visit our Internet site at http://www.gale.com

LIBRARY OF CONGRESS CATALOGING-IN-PUBLICATION DATA

Sheen, Barbara.
 Flu / by Barbara Sheen.
   p. cm. — (Diseases and disorders)
 Includes bibliographical references and index.
 Contents: What is influenza?—Flu symptoms, diagnosis, and treatment—Preventing influenza—Influenza pandemics—Preparing for the next flu pandemic.
 ISBN 1-59018-675-3 (hard cover : alk. paper) 1. Influenza—Juvenile literature. I. Title. II. Series: Diseases and disorders series.
RC150.S44 2006
616.2'03—dc22

                                                        2006009660

Printed in the United States

Table of Contents

"The Most Difficult Puzzles Ever Devised"

Charles Best, one of the pioneers in the search for a cure for diabetes, once explained what it is about medical research that intrigued him so. "It's not just the gratification of knowing one is helping people," he confided, "although that probably is a more heroic and selfless motivation. Those feelings may enter in, but truly, what I find best is the feeling of going toe to toe with nature, of trying to solve the most difficult puzzles ever devised. The answers are there somewhere, those keys that will solve the puzzle and make the patient well. But how will those keys be found?"

Since the dawn of civilization, nothing has so puzzled people— and often frightened them, as well—as the onset of illness in a body or mind that had seemed healthy before. A seizure, the inability of a heart to pump, the sudden deterioration of muscle tone in a small child—being unable to reverse such conditions or even to understand why they occur was unspeakably frustrating to healers. Even before there were names for such conditions, even before they were understood at all, each was a reminder of how complex the human body was, and how vulnerable.

While our grappling with understanding diseases has been frustrating at times, it has also provided some of humankind's most heroic accomplishments. Alexander Fleming's accidental discovery in 1928 of a mold that could be turned into penicillin has resulted in the saving of untold millions of lives. The isolation of the enzyme insulin has reversed what was once a death sentence for anyone with diabetes. There have been great strides in combating conditions for which there is not yet a cure, too. Medicines can help AIDS patients live longer, diagnostic tools such as mammography and ultrasounds can help doctors find tumors while they are treatable, and laser surgery techniques have made the most intricate, minute operations routine.

This "toe-to-toe" competition with diseases and disorders is even more remarkable when seen in a historical continuum. An astonishing amount of progress has been made in a very short time. Just two hundred years ago, the existence of germs as a cause of some diseases was unknown. In fact, it was less than 150 years ago that a British surgeon named Joseph Lister had difficulty persuading his fellow doctors that washing their hands before delivering a baby might increase the chances of a healthy delivery (especially if they had just attended to a diseased patient)!

Each book in Lucent's Diseases and Disorders series explores a disease or disorder and the knowledge that has been accumulated (or discarded) by doctors through the years. Each book also examines the tools used for pinpointing a diagnosis, as well as the various means that are used to treat or cure a disease. Finally, new ideas are presented—techniques or medicines that may be on the horizon.

Frustration and disappointment are still part of medicine, for not every disease or condition can be cured or prevented. But the limitations of knowledge are being pushed outward constantly; the "most difficult puzzles ever devised" are finding challengers every day.

An Underrated Problem

Considering the infinite variety in human lives—in geography, in working and living conditions, in habits and practices—it may be hard to think of specific experiences that all people have in common besides birth and death. One less obvious shared human experience, however, is truly universal: At some point in their lives, virtually everyone contracts influenza, or flu, as the disease is commonly known. Indeed, every person in the world is a potential flu victim and has been for thousands of years. According to reports by the ancient Greek physician Hippocrates, for example, flu has been sickening people since at least 412 B.C.

The flu virus is among the most contagious and easily transmitted pathogens. It exists in many strains and can originate anywhere, so outbreaks are difficult to prevent or predict. Just one infected individual can quickly spread the disease to hundreds of other people, so it is hard to control; between 5 and 15 percent of the world's population contracts influenza each and every year.

Not Just a Seasonal Nuisance

Despite the disease's infectious nature, influenza is not taken seriously enough. Many people incorrectly think of the flu as a seasonal nuisance that is no more debilitating than the common cold. Explains influenza expert Arno Karlen: "We simply fail to regard influenza with the degree of seriousness it deserves; we shrug, we confuse it with the common cold, and we talk about 'a flu bug going around' as if it were no more than the viral equivalent of an itch or a scratch."[1]

In reality, the influenza virus is powerful and potentially lethal. It makes its victims feel so sick that those who do not take flu seriously are often shocked by the diagnosis. According to Dr. Neil Schachter, director of respiratory care at New York's Mount Sinai School of Medicine, that is what happened

A young man suffers chills from the flu—a common, highly contagious, and sometimes serious illness.

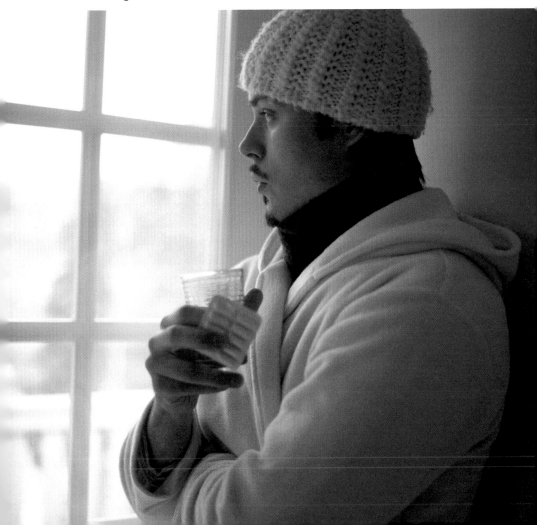

to a woman named Coop: "After a weeklong bout of cough and high fever that left her, in her own words, 'too exhausted to talk,' Coop dragged herself into the ER, convinced she had a rare deadly disease. She was stunned to hear that she had the flu, the same flu that was affecting millions of Americans."[2]

The World Health Organization (WHO) reports that approximately 3 to 5 million people worldwide are hospitalized with the ailment each year, and 250,000 to 500,000 die from flu-related complications such as pneumonia and respiratory or heart failure. In the United States alone, the flu sends an estimated 250,000 people to the hospital annually and results in about 36,000 deaths. And 5 to 10 percent of all flu-related hospitalizations have fatal outcomes.

Not only that, flu can worsen chronic health problems. For instance, because influenza affects the respiratory tract, it stimulates asthma attacks in asthma sufferers. Individuals with symptoms of congestive heart failure often experience worsening of that condition due to the flu.

Economic and Social Costs

Fortunately, most flu cases do not lead to hospitalization or death. Still, influenza is an incapacitating illness that makes people take to their beds for anywhere from a few days to more than a week, causing enormous economic and social consequences. Take, for example, Brooklyn resident Marilyn's description of her son's family: "Five of them came down with the flu. Between all five, they must have gone to the doctor at least eight times. The three children were out of school for about 14 days in all and my son missed a day and a half of work. Since he owns a business, his being out affected a lot of other people."[3] In fact, according to the Centers for Disease Control and Prevention (CDC), an estimated 20 million school days are missed each year in the United States due to the flu. During seasonal flu outbreaks, it is not uncommon for average school absentee rates to double. Since teachers are unlikely to introduce new concepts when too many students are missing, this directly impacts the learning process.

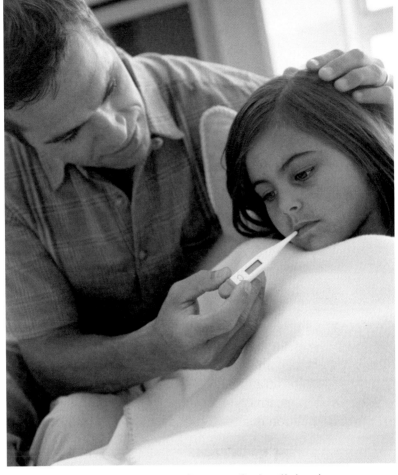

A father takes time off from work to care for his ill daughter. Absences from work to care for sick family members are a regular occurrence.

Sick children also affect the workforce. According to the U.S. Department of Labor, four-fifths of all mothers with school-age children are in the paid labor force. When children fall ill at school, working parents must leave the workplace to take sick children home, where they often stay in order to care for the ailing child.

That is not the only way influenza depletes the labor force. Ten to 12 percent of all workplace absenteeism is caused by the illness. This translates to a cost of $7 billion annually in paid sick days. Other workers lose their wages entirely: Forty percent of all hourly workers in the United States are not paid for sick time off. This adds up to more than $13 billion in lost earnings and decreased productivity.

Sick workers who come to work but are too ill to do their jobs effectively also decrease productivity as well as spread the virus to coworkers. This ultimately results in more absenteeism. Moreover, many people suffer from fatigue for as long as three weeks after flu symptoms disappear. Although these workers appear fully recovered, their ability to perform at optimal levels may be compromised.

The medical costs of flu are also phenomenal. According to the U.S. Department of Health and Human Services, the annual outlay of flu-linked doctor and hospital visits totals between $1 billion and $3 billion, depending on the extent of the outbreak. This figure does not include the price of prescription or over-the-counter medications. Nor does it take into account the rising health-care costs due to flu-related medical claims to businesses that provide workers with health insurance.

Moreover, all of these costs are based on an average seasonal flu outbreak. In years when heavier-than-normal flu outbreaks occur, these numbers rise significantly. And when a global outbreak, or pandemic, strikes, fatalities and social and economic costs skyrocket.

Importance of Knowledge

In light of the significant effects influenza has on society, it is unreasonable and dangerous to dismiss influenza as a minor problem. By learning more about the flu, how it is spread, how it is treated, what dangers it poses, and how it can be prevented, individuals can help not only themselves and their loved ones, but society in general. Such knowledge could decrease flu outbreaks, thereby reducing flu-related deaths as well as limiting the economic and social impact of the illness.

CHAPTER ONE

What Is Influenza?

Influenza, or flu, is an acute, highly contagious infection of the respiratory tract that affects the nose, throat, and large airways of the lungs. It is characterized by sometimes severe fever, congestion, sore throat, and muscle ache.

A virus causes influenza. Viruses are microscopic parasites that invade the body, interfere with normal body functions, and often cause disease. So small that millions can fit on the head of a pin, viruses are responsible for dozens of illnesses, including chicken pox, hepatitis, acquired immunodeficiency syndrome (AIDS), and the common cold, to name just a few, as well as influenza.

The influenza virus consists of strands of the genetic material ribonucleic acid (RNA) encased in a protective capsule made of two proteins, hemagglutinin and neuraminidase. The proteins give the virus its shape, while the RNA carries the information needed for the organism to replicate itself. Replication is all a virus does, but viruses are not independent living organisms—they cannot reproduce on their own. Consequently, the influenza virus must get inside a living cell within another organism to multiply.

Viruses enter the human body through bodily fluids, in food or water, and, as is the case of the flu virus, via inhalation and/or physical contact. Once in the body, the virus attaches itself to host cells by its proteins. Like matching jigsaw puzzle pieces, the shape of the proteins on the flu virus matches that of receptors on respiratory tract cells, which is why the influenza virus invades that part of the body.

Once attached, the virus burrows into the cell and uses nutrients from the cell to reproduce. This prevents the host cell from performing its normal function and eventually destroys it. Once the cell can no longer supply the nutrients the virus needs, the replicated viruses burst out of the cell and infect other healthy cells. "In essence," explains author and influenza expert Pete Davies, "it's a destructive form of molecular burglary; flu gets into the building, cracks the safe, takes what it wants, and wrecks the place on its way out."[4]

It takes about ten hours from the time a flu virus enters a cell until it bursts out. In this time, between one hundred thousand and 1 million new virus particles are formed, each of which is capable of destroying even more cells and producing more masses of viruses. "Viruses are the terrorists of the microbial world. Relentless, secretive, and lethal, they are focused on a single purpose—finding new living cells to attack and destroy,"[5] states Neil Schachter.

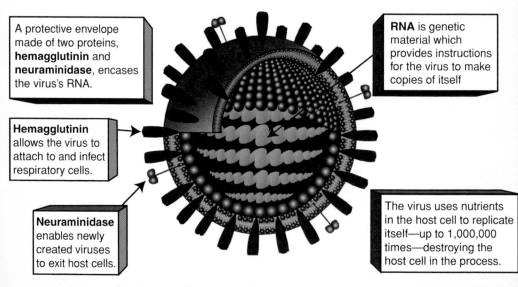

The Flu Virus

Flu viruses enter the body through inhalation. Although they contain genetic materials (RNA), they cannot reproduce on their own, but must enter another living cell in order to replicate.

A protective envelope made of two proteins, **hemagglutinin** and **neuraminidase**, encases the virus's RNA.

RNA is genetic material which provides instructions for the virus to make copies of itself

Hemagglutinin allows the virus to attach to and infect respiratory cells.

The virus uses nutrients in the host cell to replicate itself—up to 1,000,000 times—destroying the host cell in the process.

Neuraminidase enables newly created viruses to exit host cells.

Proteins give the virus its shape, while RNA carries the information needed for the virus to replicate.

Recognizing Surface Proteins

As soon as the healthy immune system detects the presence of a flu virus, it launches a counterattack. White blood cells rush to the area. When they come in contact with a flu virus they engulf it, causing bits of the virus's surface proteins to stick to the cells. This alerts the immune system to the identity of the invader.

If the immune system has previously been exposed to these proteins, known as antigens, it releases other proteins known as antibodies. Antibodies are shaped to match a specific antigen, which they recognize, lock onto, and destroy. If, on the other hand, the immune system has never been exposed to an antigen, it takes about two weeks of exposure before the proper antibodies can be manufactured.

Thereafter, that antigen cannot harm the body. Consequently, once an individual has been infected with a virus, that person should be immune to future infections. But since there are multiple kinds of flu viruses that have the ability to change structure, or mutate, this is not the case when it comes to the flu.

Different Types of Influenza Viruses

Scientists have identified over five thousand different viruses, including three types that cause influenza. These are known as influenza virus types A, B, and C. Type A is the most virulent form of the virus, causing epidemics, which are widespread local and national outbreaks, and pandemics, which are global flu outbreaks that usually occur in repeated waves over the course of a year, causing infection in thousands of localities simultaneously. Type A infects birds, humans, and other mammals such as pigs. Types B and C are found only in humans. Type B causes illness but is usually not as harmful as type A. Type C rarely causes symptoms.

Scientists further categorize type A viruses into subtypes, or strains, according to the structure and composition of the two proteins on their surface. Hemagglutinin occurs in sixteen slightly different shapes, and neuraminidase in nine; possible combinations of these yield a total of 144 influenza A subtypes. To distinguish between them, scientists label type A viruses

The Influenza Virus

A flu virus can be round, elongated, or irregularly shaped. Inside, it contains eight segments of the genetic material RNA. Outside, the virus is enclosed in a protein envelope made of hemagglutinin, which allows the virus to attach to and infect respiratory cells, and neuraminidase, which allows newly formed viruses to exit host cells.

The RNA core provides the virus with instructions for making copies of itself. The enzyme that copies RNA does not have the ability to recognize itself. Therefore, when the flu virus replicates, errors in the new cells are not corrected. In some cases, the new viruses do not survive. In other cases, according to University of Kansas microbiology professor John C. Brown,

> The errors won't lead to anything much, except that the organism may behave a little differently, or, may "look" a little (or a lot) differently. It is the behavior and "look" differences that are a problem for us.

> When a particular influenza virus replicates the RNA genetic material many, many times . . . , errors appear. The individual virus among the group, which has the errors, now may "look" very different from the rest of the group. This virus, however, is still an influenza virus, with all the properties of such a virus; however, now there exists a new strain of influenza virus.

John C. Brown, "The Flu Is a Bummer," JBrown. http://people.ku.edu/~jbrown/ flu.html.

with names such as H1N1, H2N2, H3N2, and so on. To further differentiate between viruses, scientists often refer to flu viruses by the geographic location in which the first outbreak of the virus occurred. For example, H3N2 is also known as Hong Kong virus H3N2 or the Hong Kong Flu.

Antigenic Drift and Shift

Type A and B flu viruses change the shape or composition of their surface proteins when they replicate. This makes it difficult, or even impossible, for antibodies to lock onto them. As a result, a person can be infected with the flu repeatedly. University of Kansas microbiologist John C. Brown provides this explanation:

> If we become infected with a new viral strain, our bodies have never, ever, seen this particular "looking" virus before. Consequently, our immune system must start fresh to respond to the infections. An analogy would be that our immune system has had no previous "practice" in responding to this virus. The response is therefore relatively slow—may take many days to mount an effective response—thus, by this time, we may be very, very ill.[6]

This viral change happens in one of two ways. The more gradual, subtle way is called antigenic drift. Antigenic drift occurs constantly, causing small changes in type A and B viruses. Such changes occur because RNA has no way to check for errors as the virus makes copies of itself. At first, the errors may

Spiky surface proteins, visible in this computer-enhanced illustration of a flu virus, change shape when the virus replicates.

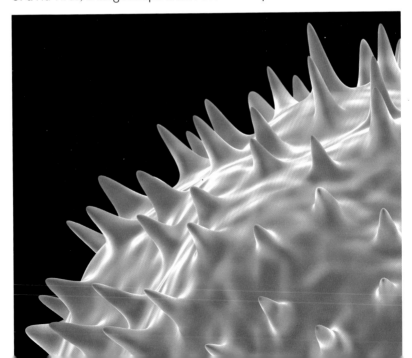

The Respiratory System

When a person inhales, air enters through the nose or the mouth. The air travels to the upper part of the throat, called the pharynx, then into the larynx, or voice box. From here, the air passes through the windpipe, or trachea. The trachea branches into two tubes known as the bronchi, or bronchial tubes, that carry air into the lungs. The bronchi branch into smaller and smaller tubes called bronchioles. These end in tiny air sacs called alveoli. Capillaries surround the alveoli. Oxygen passes from the alveoli to the capillaries, where it is exchanged for carbon dioxide. The carbon dioxide is then exhaled.

Since bacteria, viruses, and other foreign particles are often transmitted by air, cilia, tiny hairs that line the mucous membranes in the nose, mouth, throat, and bronchi, help protect the lungs from infection. Cilia wave back and forth, trapping foreign particles in the sticky mucous membranes. The foreign particles are then expelled through the mouth or destroyed by acids in the digestive system. But not all foreign particles are trapped by the cilia. These settle in the nose, throat, and lungs, causing disease.

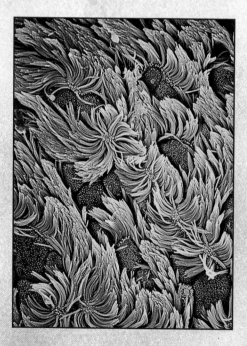

A colored electron micrograph shows cilia lining the nasal cavity. The hairlike structures help protect the lungs from infection.

be so minor that the immune system can still recognize the virus and defend itself. But gradually, as the modified viruses continue to replicate and change, the shape of their surface proteins alters just enough to make it difficult for antibodies to lock onto them. When this happens, heavier-than-normal flu outbreaks follow. Author and influenza expert John M. Barry describes this phenomenon in this manner:

> One way to conceptualize antigenic drift is to think of a football player wearing a uniform with white pants, a green shirt, and a white helmet with a green V emblazoned on it. The immune system can recognize that uniform instantly and attack it. If the uniform changes slightly—if, for example, a green stripe is added to the white pants while everything else remains the same—the immune system will continue to recognize the virus with little difficulty. But if the uniform goes from a green shirt and white pants to a white shirt and green pants, the immune system may not recognize the virus easily.[7]

Antigenic shift is a more abrupt and major change. It occurs only in type A viruses and is responsible for large-scale flu epidemics and pandemics. It occurs when two different flu viruses come together and exchange or reassort their surface proteins. This creates a new influenza A subtype whose shape bears little resemblance to the original viruses and is, therefore, unrecognizable to the immune system. It is, according to Barry, "the equivalent of the virus changing from a green shirt and white pants to an orange shirt and black pants."[8] Consequently, people have no protection against the new virus.

A Communicable Disease

No matter how much the structure of the flu virus varies, all influenza viruses are contagious. The virus is transmitted from person to person on tiny respiratory droplets that form when an infected individual sheds the virus by coughing or sneezing. Uninfected individuals then breathe in the droplets, or the

Getting the Flu

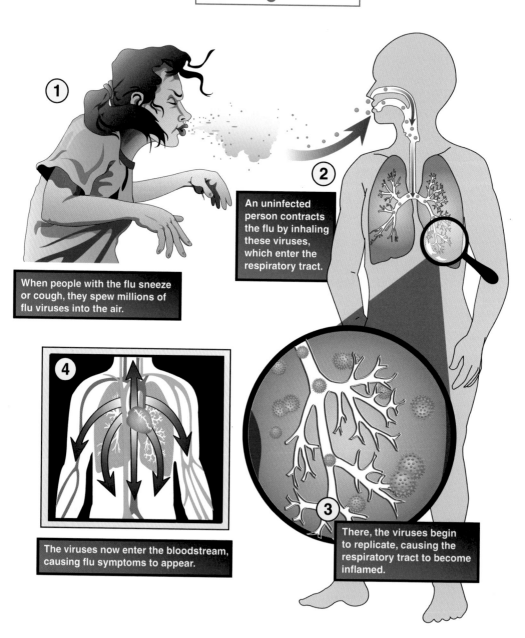

① When people with the flu sneeze or cough, they spew millions of flu viruses into the air.

② An uninfected person contracts the flu by inhaling these viruses, which enter the respiratory tract.

③ There, the viruses begin to replicate, causing the respiratory tract to become inflamed.

④ The viruses now enter the bloodstream, causing flu symptoms to appear.

droplets may land directly on an individual's eyes or other exposed mucous membranes in the nose or mouth. Millions of flu viruses can be carried on one droplet, which can linger in the air from an hour to a day and still infect a person. Consequently, a person can be infected with a flu virus from someone who sneezed hours ago. And since a sneeze travels out of the lungs at approximately 100 miles per hour (150km/h), each droplet can travel 3 feet (1m) and affect a wide area.

Touching a surface that is infected with the virus, then touching one's mouth or nose also spreads the virus. For example, if an infected person coughs or sneezes onto a computer keyboard and another person touches the keyboard, then rubs his or her nose, that person will become infected. In an interview with ABC News, Marie Kassai, a registered nurse and an infection control professional, explains: "People wipe their faces, they blow their noses, they cough into their hands and then they shake hands or touch other areas."[9]

Moreover, since the virus can linger on hard surfaces and cause infection for up to two days, infection can be spread in this manner for extended periods. John, a librarian, talks about his concerns:

> In my library, I'm always afraid of sneezers. Second worst are coughers, especially people who don't cover their mouths and let germs launch like missiles. From what I know about germs, I know that they are everywhere—from the books, to the tabletops, to the computer keyboards, and especially the circulation desk, where library patrons put their hands and sometimes sneeze right at you. Outside of wearing a mask, what can you do in a public setting like this where we're supposed to be patron friendly? The worst part is the germs don't go away when the sneezers and coughers leave. They can sneeze on a book in the morning and a few hours later, you unknowingly handle the book; it's no wonder so many librarians come down with the flu every year.[10]

Making matters worse, the virus can be spread by individuals who have yet to exhibit signs of infection as well as by individuals who appear to be over the illness. Infected individuals can spread the virus for seven to ten days, including twenty-four hours before recognizable symptoms appear and up to four days after symptoms are gone.

Conditions That Enhance Transmission

Because of the way the virus is transmitted, flu outbreaks are most likely to occur in conditions in which people are in close contact. This helps explain why flu outbreaks occur year-round in warm climate regions of developing nations in Asia and Africa, where people live in constantly crowded conditions, and why outbreaks are concentrated in the late fall to early spring in other parts of the world where seasonal cold weather forces people to spend more time crowded together indoors. Lack of proper ventilation keeps the virus contained and hastens the spread at any time of year.

Places like crowded malls, commuter trains, airplanes, sports arenas, movie theaters, offices, crowded elevators, nursing homes, day-care centers, college dormitories, and schools provide excellent environments for the virus to spread. Indeed, schools are such good places for the virus to spread that one-third of all family members in which there is at least one school-age child becomes infected with the flu each year. In fact, many health-care professionals say that if one sibling in a family contracts the flu, it is almost inevitable that other siblings will come down with the illness, too. Marilyn describes how the flu spread in her son's family:

> There are six people in my son's family, and five of them came down with the flu this year. First my eleven-year-old grandson got sick. The flu was going around his middle school and he picked it up there. Then, two days later my eight-year-old grandson started running a fever. He caught it from his brother. Then, my daughter-in-law started coughing and feeling badly. By the time the eleven-year-old

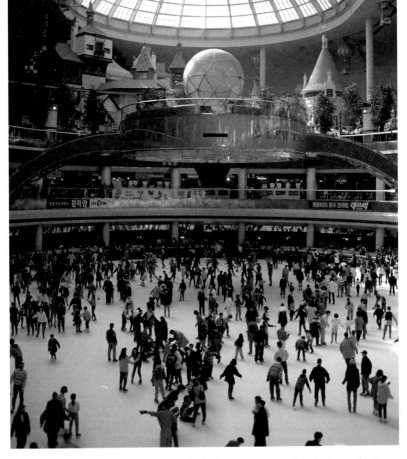

Flu germs spread easily in crowded places such as this indoor skating rink at a Japanese shopping mall.

went back to school, the baby was sick. Then my son came down with it. My daughter-in-law wound up with bronchitis, and the baby developed pneumonia. The only one who didn't get sick was my oldest grandson. He's a teenager and doesn't spend that much time with his brothers. Maybe that saved him.[11]

Because influenza is so easily transmitted, outbreaks can very quickly become epidemics or pandemics. Anyone, no matter an individual's gender, age, or ethnic background, can be infected. WHO estimates that 5 to 15 percent of the world's population contract the flu annually. It is difficult to come up with an exact number, since people in developing nations are less likely to seek medical help due to poverty or limited access to health care. Their cases, therefore, are underreported.

Percentages are highest in nations with accessible health care. The CDC estimates that as many as 20 percent of all Americans become infected each year, while Health Canada puts that number as high as 25 percent of all Canadians. Indeed, it is not uncommon for as many as one-half the population of a community to contract the illness during local outbreaks. For example, a flu outbreak in Arizona caused a reported 388 cases during the week of December 25, 2005. It affected so many people that the emergency room staff of Scottsdale Healthcare Osborn Hospital reported seeing more than 200 patients per day, double the usual number. "We have been slammed,"[12] declared Nancy Neff, a spokeswoman for Banner Desert Medical Center in Mesa, another area hospital that was hard-hit.

A friendly nurse discusses medication with an elderly patient. The elderly are particularly susceptible to the flu virus.

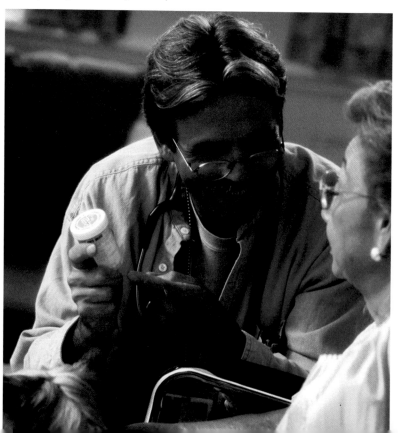

People at Greater Risk

Clearly, once the flu virus begins circulating, it is hard to avoid. But certain people are more vulnerable to infection than others. Individuals in this group are also more likely to develop serious complications such as pneumonia, bronchitis, and fluid in the lungs, all of which affect their ability to breathe and can therefore be fatal. These individuals have one thing in common—a weakened immune system. They include people age sixty-five and older, children ages six to twenty-three months, pregnant women, and individuals with diseases that compromise the immune system.

The elderly are among the most vulnerable group. The immune system weakens with age and may not work as effectively as it does in younger persons. Thus, elderly people are often less able to fight off the virus and more likely to develop a secondary infection such as pneumonia. In the United States, 90 percent of flu-related deaths, about twenty thousand annually, occur among this group. In addition, some groups of elderly individuals are at even higher risk, such as residents of nursing homes or other long-term care facilities who share a common residence. Flu outbreaks have been known to sweep through these facilities.

People who are eighty-five years old or older are especially vulnerable. According to the American Geriatrics Association, they are sixteen times more likely to die of an influenza-related death than people aged sixty-five to sixty-nine. Marilyn, whose grandfather was in this group, recalls: "My grandfather was 86 when he died. He came down with the flu and was very sick, much sicker than most people with the flu. We did everything we could to take care of him, but he was too old and weak. The virus got into his lungs and he got pneumonia. That's what killed him."[13]

Young Children

Young children between six and twenty-three months of age are another susceptible group. Before age two, children's immune systems are not fully developed, and their lungs are not as strong as those of older children and adults. Moreover, young children are likely to put their hands in their mouths or rub their noses after touching infected surfaces. This age group is two to three times more likely to contract the flu than older children and adults. They are hospitalized just as often as the elderly due to flu-related complications but are less likely to die.

According to the National Foundation of Infectious Diseases, in the United States, about ninety-two children two years old or less die each year as a result of flu-associated illnesses. Regan, whose son came close to death, describes his experience: "My then ten month old son developed the flu and was subsequently hospitalized after exhibiting symptoms of respiratory distress [difficulty breathing]. Within 24 hours of his admission he went into respiratory failure . . . developed double pneumonia and a staph infection of the lung, was on a ventilator and suffered through more crises than I care to recall. He was hospitalized for three weeks. He did survive."[14]

Other Risks

No matter what age, people with chronic heart or respiratory diseases such as asthma and other diseases such as cancer, AIDS, and diabetes are also at risk. These illnesses compromise the immune system, making affected individuals less able to fight off infection. For the same reason, individuals suffering from malnutrition are also in danger. According to WHO, poorly nourished populations are more likely to contract the flu and develop serious complications than well-nourished groups.

In order to prevent the developing fetus from being attacked as a foreign invader, a pregnant woman's immune system is somewhat suppressed. This makes her vulnerable to infection and complications. According to Dr. Neil Silverman of Cedars-Sinai Medical Center in Los Angeles, "Women who suffer an influenza infection during pregnancy, particularly in the third trimester, are at high risk for developing serious complications that can impact their health and that of the baby."[15]

Health-care workers who are in direct contact with influenza patients are susceptible to infection, although not

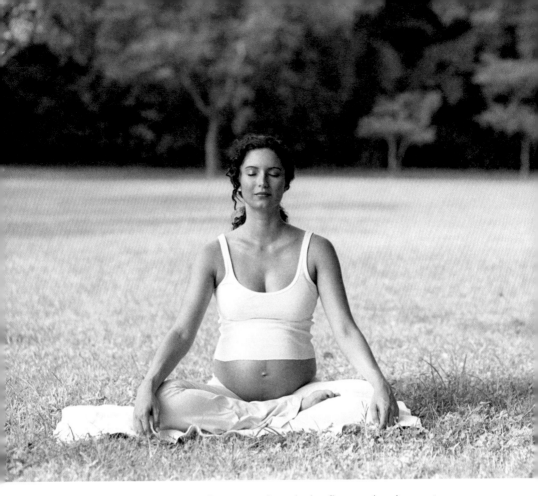

A pregnant woman who gets sick with the flu can develop serious health problems—both for her and the baby.

likely to develop complications. Doctors and nurses as well as hospital and nursing-home staff all fall into this group. Caregivers in day-care centers are also at risk. Marie Kassai explains: "One of the populations where the spread of infection is most difficult to contain is in a daycare center. You have children who have runny noses, who don't really understand how to contain infection."[16]

It is clear that although the virus is most likely to infect those who are most vulnerable, anyone can contract the flu. Since flu viruses change so often, even the hardiest individuals can become infected repeatedly. That is why flu outbreaks sicken millions of people around the world each year. For those most at risk of developing complications, the results can be deadly.

CHAPTER TWO

Flu Symptoms, Diagnosis, and Treatment

Infection with the influenza virus causes specific symptoms. Medical professionals base their diagnosis on the presence of these symptoms and the prevalence of flu in the area. Even when a diagnosis is made, however, treatment options are limited. There is no known medication that can cure the flu. Available treatments can lessen flu symptoms, make patients feel more comfortable, and decrease the risk of complications developing.

When Symptoms Arise

When the flu virus enters the body, it settles in the mucous membranes of the nose, sinuses, throat, bronchial tubes, and sometimes the lungs. What we think of as flu symptoms are the result of both the virus itself and the body's reaction to the virus. For example, viral damage to infected cells and the release of inflammatory chemicals provoke the immune system to release its own inflammatory substances that cause swelling, redness, heat, and pain in response to the antigens.

When flu virus particles burst out of destroyed cells, powerful inflammatory proteins called cytokines spill into the body.

Cytokines irritate the nerves in the throat and airways, which produces coughing. Coughing is also a way for the body to expel the virus. Flu patients complain of frequent bone-jarring coughs that many sufferers say is the worst symptom of the illness. "I was coughing a lot," Sammy, a boy who contracted the flu in 2006, recalls. "The coughing made my chest hurt and feel tight. It was worse when I first woke up, I'd cough so [much] for so long that I had trouble getting air into my body."[17]

Cytokines also trigger a rise in body temperature. Since viruses cannot replicate at high temperatures, development of fever is an important defense mechanism. Flu patients typically develop a fever between 102°F (38.89°C) and 104°F (40°C). Fever can last from three to four days, sometimes longer, and is usually accompanied by chills. Sammy's brother, Liam, who also contracted the flu, remembers: "I felt horrible. I had a high fever for roughly a week. It ranged from 101 to 104 degrees [38°C to 40°C]."[18]

A person who is sick with flu might experience severe bouts of coughing, which is one method the body uses to expel the virus.

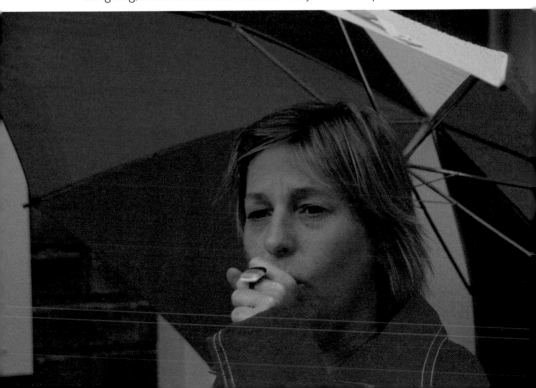

The presence of cytokines also elicits a reaction from nerve endings throughout the body, which, in combination with increased production of white blood cells in an infected individual's bone marrow, causes intense body aches. "I hurt all over," Liam continues. "Every part of me ached and was sensitive. My legs were the worst. I could barely walk down a flight of stairs. I just wanted to lay still without moving a muscle."[19]

Feelings of weakness and fatigue so extreme that many individuals do not have the strength to get out of bed generally accompany body pain. Although other flu symptoms usually disappear in five to seven days, lack of energy often persists for two to three weeks. That is what happened to Sammy: "I felt very tired. I was in bed for three days and I slept almost the whole day, every day. When I got out of bed to go to the bathroom, I felt so weak that I was afraid I would fall down. All I wanted to do was lie back down in my bed. Even when I went back to school I was still tired for a while."[20]

Weakness, headaches, and extreme fatigue show on the face of a woman who suffers from the flu.

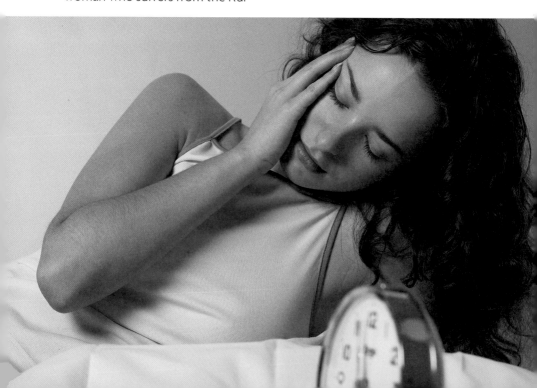

To accelerate blood flow to infected cells, other inflammatory substances known as histamines produce swelling in the mucous membranes and blood vessels lining the nose, sinuses, and throat. This causes the airways to narrow and flu sufferers to experience feelings of fullness or congestion and difficulty breathing.

In addition, the swollen membranes press against nerve endings in the throat, causing throat pain. Damage by the virus, which strips the throat raw as it destroys throat cells, intensifies this pain. Patients complain of a burning in their throat and difficulty swallowing.

Similarly, swollen membranes compress nerve endings in the sinuses, producing headaches. At the same time, in an effort to expel the virus, histamines stimulate mucus production, causing a nasal drip and frequent sneezing. Sammy remembers: "My head hurt the whole time I was sick and I was a little dizzy. My nose was running a lot. I was sneezing all the time. I used up a box of tissues a day."[21]

Making a Diagnosis

When patients complain of flu-like symptoms, in order to make an accurate diagnosis, health-care professionals examine the patient, checking for signs of fever and inflammation. A local flu outbreak is also a good indicator that the patient has contracted the flu.

Finally, because flu symptoms are similar to those of the common cold, medical providers look at the severity and presence of particular symptoms to distinguish between the two illnesses. For example, cold symptoms come on gradually, whereas the flu is characterized by a swift and sudden onset. Rob Hicks, a medical expert for the British Broadcasting System's Health Web site, which is dedicated to making the public aware of various health issues, describes the flu's onset in this way: "One minute you're happy at work, the next you . . . are too ill to do anything."[22]

Severe body aches and fever always accompany the flu, but are rarely associated with colds. When fever is linked to colds, it does not reach the high spikes associated with influenza. Other symptoms such as fatigue, coughing, sneezing, and a sore throat characterize both illnesses. But those that go with a cold are milder and less debilitating than those linked to flu. Although individuals who have a cold may feel tired, they are still able to perform their normal activities, while flu-related fatigue is so intense that individuals are forced to take to their beds. Indeed, flu symptoms are always more extreme than those of the common cold. "A cold can be annoying and depressing, but you still have the energy to complain," notes Neil Schachter. "In a flu you often feel too miserable to talk. The fever, body aches, and bone-jarring cough make you weak and ill. Once you have had a full-blown flu, it is likely that you will know when it has struck again."[23]

Antiviral Medications

People diagnosed with the flu often mistakenly think antibiotic medications will cure their symptoms. But antibiotics, which destroy bacteria, have no effect on viruses. Flu treatment, therefore, involves relieving the discomfort or shortening the duration of flu symptoms. Such treatment makes the flu easier to endure and lessens the risk of complications arising.

Two antiviral drugs—Tamiflu, which is known generically as oseltamivir, and Relenza, also known as zanamivir—are often prescribed. Both reduce the duration of flu symptoms by about 30 percent. These medications work by inhibiting the virus's ability to escape from infected cells. As a result, the immune system lessens its reaction, and symptoms linked to the inflammatory response diminish.

Since these medications are not specific to a particular strain of flu, they can be used to combat new influenza subtypes whenever they arise. To be effective, both medications must be taken within the first forty-eight hours that flu symptoms appear. Thereafter, the presence of the virus elicits too large an inflammatory response for antiviral medications to control. Tamiflu is administered orally. Relenza is inhaled through a breath-activated plastic device that resembles an asthma inhaler.

Although both medications usually help people feel better and resume their normal activities sooner, as with all medications there are risks of side effects. Relenza can irritate the airways and cause wheezing and other breathing problems, particularly in children, and is not administered to patients under age twelve. Tamiflu can cause diarrhea, vomiting, and abdominal pain, but such side effects are rare.

Despite the benefits of antiviral drugs, some health-care professionals advocate limiting their use. Their concern is not the risk of side effects, but rather the possibility that repeated exposure to antiviral medications could cause flu viruses to develop resistance to the drugs. Indeed, the H3N2 virus that circulated during the 2005–2006 flu season developed resistance to two other antiviral medicines, amantadine and flumadine. If a future flu pandemic arises, scientists are counting on Tamiflu and Relenza to help contain it. Widespread resistance to these drugs in the absence of effective alternatives could have tragic consequences.

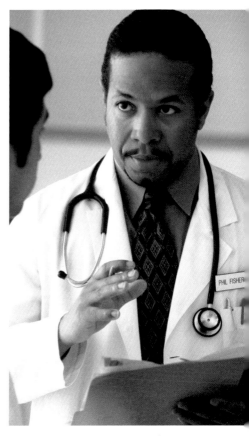

Some doctors recommend limited use of antiviral medications, fearing that over-use could enable flu viruses to develop resistance to the drugs.

Nevertheless, for those individuals at risk of developing flu-related complications, antiviral drugs are invaluable. They have been shown to cut the risk of developing complications and can therefore save lives.

Bed Rest and Fluids

Whether or not an antiviral medication is administered, all flu patients are directed to rest and drink plenty of fluids. The body uses a great deal of energy to fight the flu. Getting adequate rest strengthens the body, supports the immune system, and promotes healing. "Experts agree that the best thing you can do for . . . the flu is to stay home and stay off your feet. Hide under the covers or camp out in your Barcalounger,"[24] recommends health writer Joan Morris.

Replacing fluids lost due to fever is also essential. Without adequate fluids, patients are at risk of becoming dehydrated.

Drinking hot tea several times a day can ease flu symptoms by reducing coughing and facilitating the release of mucus from the nose and lungs.

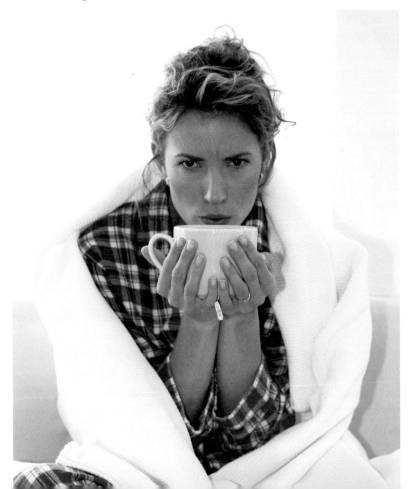

Dehydration is characterized by excessive thirst, inability to urinate, lethargy, confusion, and irrational behavior. Severe dehydration can lead to shock and death.

Drinking liquids also thins and loosens mucus in the upper respiratory tract. Flu patients are advised to consume at least sixty-four ounces (1.89l) of liquids a day. Water, fruit juices, noncarbonated sports drinks, and broth are all recommended for this purpose. Milk, which contains substances that stimulate mucus production, and caffeinated beverages are not suggested. Caffeine constricts blood vessels in the respiratory tract, making breathing more difficult. And because caffeine is a stimulant, it interferes with an individual's ability to rest.

With that said, it is interesting to note that medical professionals often advise flu patients to drink tea. Although it contains caffeine, it has other properties that ease flu symptoms. Tea contains chemicals that dilate the bronchial tubes, reducing coughing. Adding honey and lemon to tea soothes the throat, while inhaling vapors from tea or other hot liquids thins mucus and speeds up mucus release from the nose and lungs. "I recommend three to four cups of hot tea throughout the day when you come down with a respiratory infection," advises Neil Schachter. "I urge coffee drinkers to switch to tea for the duration of their symptoms."[25]

Cold liquids, too, can be useful. They numb a sore throat and are absorbed by the body quickly. In addition, most sports drinks replace essential electrolytes like sodium lost due to fever. "I drank a lot of cold Gatorade," Liam notes. "It felt good on my throat, gave me more fluids, and helped raise my energy level."[26]

Over-the-Counter Remedies

Some patients turn to over-the-counter remedies to help ease their symptoms. These include pain relievers, saline nasal sprays, decongestants, antihistamines, cough medicines, and menthol salves.

Pain relievers such as aspirin, acetaminophen, and ibuprofen contain chemicals that inhibit the production of cytokines.

As a result, inflammation is reduced, as is pain and fever. The use of aspirin in viral infections in children under eighteen, however, has been linked to the development of Reyes syndrome, a potentially fatal disease of the liver and brain. Therefore, experts recommend acetaminophen or ibuprofen for juvenile flu patients. That is why eleven-year-old Liam did not take aspirin: "I took Motrin [ibuprofen] or Tylenol [acetaminophen]. The Motrin helped me the most. It made the fever go down a lot, and that made me feel better. It also helped with the leg pain."[27]

Decongestants and antihistamines are also useful. They relieve congestion and reduce sneezing and nasal drip. Antihistamines inhibit the production of histamines and the resulting symptoms they cause. And because most antihistamines cause drowsiness, they help patients rest.

Decongestants shrink blood vessels in the nasal passages, which keeps the airways from being blocked and makes nasal breathing easier. However, decongestants also increase a person's blood pressure and heart rate, making them a bad choice for people with heart disease.

Saline nasal sprays also reduce nasal congestion. When they are sprayed into the nostrils, they restore moisture to nasal passages by dissolving dried and hardened mucus, which opens the airways.

Cough medicines, formally known as antitussives, are also popular. They suppress the cough center of the brain, which keeps patients from coughing and allows them to get much-needed rest. Menthol salves, which are rubbed on the chest, help ease respiratory congestion in another way, by making the body produce watery mucus that washes out the airways. Moreover, the menthol-scented fumes are soothing.

Home Remedies

Home remedies such as chicken soup, water therapy, gargling with salt water, and using a humidifier are also beneficial. Chicken soup has been used to treat flu for at least one thousand years. It has the same beneficial effects as other hot liq-

The Sauerkraut Cure

For centuries, folk healers have claimed that sauerkraut has medicinal properties. A 2005 study indicates that this theory may be correct. Sauerkraut may be an effective treatment against the avian flu, a lethal form of the flu that affects birds, humans, and other mammals.

According to an article in the *Milwaukee Journal Sentinel*, "Scientists at Seoul National University in South Korea fed an extract of kimchi, a spicy Korean variant of sauerkraut, to 13 chickens infected with avian flu, and a week later, 11 of the birds started to recover."

More studies are needed to prove that sauerkraut has a curative effect on the flu, and if so, why. In the meantime, sales of kimchi and sauerkraut have increased significantly throughout the world. It appears that many people are adding sauerkraut to their arsenal of flu treatments. Others are adding the product to their diets in the hope of preventing the flu. Even if fermented cabbage does not prove to speed flu recovery, since it is loaded with vitamins and minerals it can help individuals stay healthy.

Karen Herzog, "Meet the Chicken Soup of Avian Flu," *JSOnline*, November 3, 2005. www.jsonline.com/alive/news/nov05/367937.asp.

uids and provides a source of nutrition. And it may actually have medicinal value. A 2000 study at the University of Nebraska Medical Center in Omaha found that chicken soup contains chemicals that have an anti-inflammatory effect on the body. In this study, chicken soup was applied directly to neutrophils, white blood cells that rush to the respiratory tract and stimulate the release of mucus. The study found that the soup slowed the movement of the cells, which reduced the release of mucus and congestion. "Without a doubt there are biologically active compounds in the chicken soup that can slow neutrophil migration,"[28] says study leader Stephen Rennard.

Although more research is needed to prove that chicken soup is indeed an anti-inflammatory, many people depend on it to ease flu symptoms. Mariane, who describes herself as "a Mom dealing with a very bad flu season," relies on the soup: "I made [it] yesterday for my nine-year-old daughter who has the flu. She felt better immediately and the flu appears to have gone through her system in about 36 hours. I have been treating myself and only had one half day in bed, with very minor symptoms."[29]

Water therapy is another age-old flu treatment. A cool shower reduces fever, while applying an ice pack to inflamed sinuses reduces painful swelling. Steam produced in a hot bath or shower moistens hardened mucus and gets it flowing. A hot-mist humidifier, which disperses moisture into the air in the form of a fine steam, has the same effect. Dry air is common during cold weather, when household heating reduces humidity in the air. Overly dry air irritates the airways, worsening flu-related congestion. In addition to adding moisture to the air, most humidifiers have a special compartment in which users can add compounds such as eucalyptus oil or menthol spray, which, when they are diffused into the air with the steam, provide a soothing scent and relief from coughing. According to experts at the Mayo Clinic in Rochester, Minnesota, "A humidifier provides comfort and relief for adults and children with influenza."[30]

Gargling with warm salt water can also be effective. The saline solution rinses away virus-laden mucus in the throat. As a result, congestion and inflammation are lessened. "It provides instant and welcome relief," Schachter says, "and it may lessen the duration of the infection as you lower the amount of . . . viruses in the airways."[31]

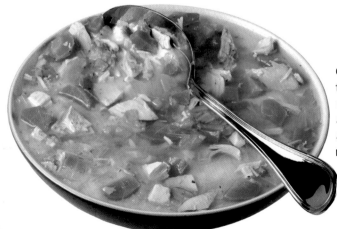

Chicken soup, long thought to be a remedy for colds and flu, may actually have some medicinal value.

The Connection Between Flu and Pneumonia

Pneumonia is a disease of the bronchioles and alveoli of the lungs and therefore affects the exchange of air. According to influenza expert John M. Barry:

> Pneumonia is almost always caused by some kind of microorganism invading the lungs, followed by an infusion of the body's infection-fighting weapons. The resulting inflamed mix of cells, enzymes, cell debris, fluid, and the equivalent of scar tissue . . . [causes] the lung, normally soft and spongy, to become firm, solid, and inelastic. The disease kills when either [this hardening] becomes so widespread that the lungs cannot transfer enough oxygen into the bloodstream, or the pathogen enters the bloodstream and carries the infection throughout the body.

Barry goes on to explain:

> Influenza causes pneumonia either directly, by a massive viral invasion of the lungs, or indirectly—and more commonly—by destroying certain parts of the body's defenses and allowing so-called secondary invaders, bacteria, to infect the lungs virtually unopposed. There is also evidence that the influenza virus makes it easier for some bacteria to invade the lung not only by generally wiping out defense mechanisms but by specifically facilitating some bacteria's ability to attach to lung tissue.

John M. Barry, *The Great Influenza*. London: Penguin, 2005.

Alternative Treatments

Some patients supplement their treatment with alternative remedies. Due to lack of conclusive proof of their safety or effectiveness and lack of standards regulating their quality,

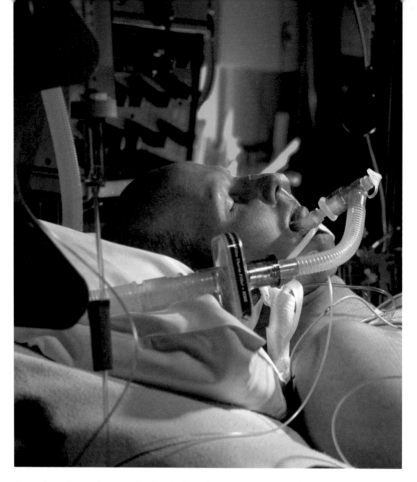

A patient breathes with the help of a respirator. Such measures may be needed when flu leads to pneumonia.

traditional medical professionals do not commonly accept alternative treatments. Yet many people say these treatments ease flu symptoms.

Elderberry juice, an herbal remedy said to have antiviral properties, has been used to treat the flu for twenty-five hundred years. Whether or not elderberries are an antiviral substance is uncertain, but a 2002 study at the University of Oslo in Norway indicated this claim may indeed be valid. An elderberry extract called Sambucol was administered to thirty flu patients within the first forty-eight hours of the appearance of symptoms, while a second group received a placebo. Ninety percent of the Sambucol group were without flu symptoms within three days, while the placebo group remained symptomatic for six days. A similar study in Israel in 2004 yielded comparable results. Scientists do not know how elderberry extract works or whether it is as effective as it appears to be, but some flu patients are adding Sambucol to their treatment. Experts warn that since parts of the plant are poisonous, individuals should be careful about the quality of the product they use.

Other alternative treatments involve the use of nutritional supplements such as zinc. Taken in the form of candy-like tablets called lozenges that slowly dissolve in the mouth, zinc is said to reduce inflammation and inhibit viral replication. Studies into zinc's medicinal properties have produced conflicting results. Still, many individuals rely on the mineral. "I pop a zinc lozenge every few hours at the first sign of infection," John explains. "It soothes my throat and makes me feel better. I know scientists don't agree on its value, but when you get the flu anything that makes you feel better and recover faster is worth a shot."[32]

Dealing with Complications

Most flu sufferers recover within ten days. But this is not always the case. If the virus penetrates too deeply into the lungs or if a secondary bacterial infection arises, causing viral or bacterial pneumonia, the results can be life threatening. Depending on the severity of the illness, patients may be hospitalized and connected to an artificial breathing machine known as a respirator. It causes the lungs to inflate and deflate automatically—in effect, breathing for the patient. But if damage to the lungs is too great, the patient may not recuperate. Currently, flu-related pneumonia is the sixth leading cause of death in the United States.

Clearly, the flu is a serious illness that causes unpleasant symptoms that take a toll on the body. Since there is no treatment that can cure the flu, individuals use a variety of remedies to ease their symptoms. And since there is no cure, health-care providers and the general public alike look for ways to avoid symptoms by preventing infection.

CHAPTER THREE

Preventing Influenza

There is no way to completely prevent flu outbreaks, especially if the virus mutates radically. There are, however, a number of measures that individuals can take to lessen the spread of the virus and to guard against the illness. Such steps minimize the size and severity of flu epidemics.

Flu Vaccines

Vaccines create immunity to particular illnesses by exposing the immune system to a small dose of greatly weakened or inactivated (dead) viruses. Such exposure stimulates the production of antibodies specific to those viruses. If the full-strength viruses invade a vaccinated person in the future, the immune system recognizes them and quickly produces the appropriate antibodies to destroy them.

Medical professionals and public health officials agree that getting a flu vaccine is the best way to prevent, or at least minimize, a person's chances of contracting the flu, thereby reducing flu outbreaks. Dr. Rex Archer, president of the National Association of County and City Health Officials, states: "The public health need is that every person in the country get a flu shot. . . . If you want to talk about being a citizen in the country and having a public responsibility and duty, we should all get a flu shot."[33]

The flu vaccine consists of two type A influenza viruses and one type B virus. For the vaccine to be most effective, scientists must closely match the vaccine viral subtypes to circulating viral strains. The components of the flu vaccine are adapted as needed, and people must be inoculated annually. Indeed, in the period between 1976 and 2006, thirty-nine changes were made to the vaccine.

Determining the composition of the vaccine is difficult and requires global collaboration. Decisions on their composition must be made nine to ten months before the flu season begins. To make an accurate determination, WHO maintains a network of 112 influenza surveillance and control centers located in eighty-three countries whose function is to monitor influenza activity and isolate circulating influenza viruses. The viral samples are identified in four collaborating research centers located in the United States, England, Japan, and Australia.

Wearing protective gear, a microbiologist at the National Center for Infectious Diseases conducts research on flu vaccines.

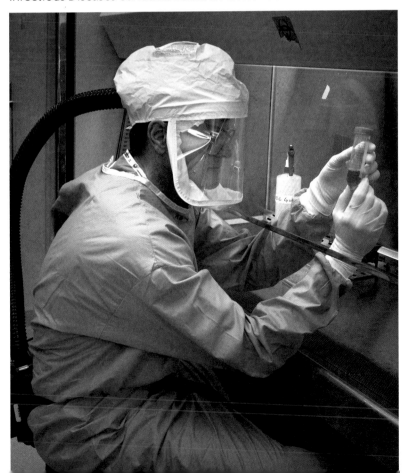

Twice a year, in February in the Northern Hemisphere and September in the Southern Hemisphere, directors of the collaborating research centers, consulting scientists, and public health officials review these findings and select the three viruses most likely to cause problems in the upcoming flu season.

Once this is done, scientists mix the viruses with a strain that is safe for humans and inject the mixture into fertilized eggs. In the next few weeks, the mixture develops into a viral strain that will stimulate the immune system to manufacture antibodies against all the incorporated strains. Using the new viral strain, pharmaceutical companies produce about 250 million doses of the vaccine for global use each year. Once enough doses are made, the vaccine is treated with chemicals that weaken or kill the viruses so that they cannot cause infection. Then the vaccine is tested for safety and purity before it is distributed to health-care providers. The process takes at least nine months.

The vaccine is generally available by October in the Northern Hemisphere and June in the Southern. It is most effective in adults and children and less effective in people over sixty-five, who have a decreased immune response.

By the time the vaccine becomes available, it is possible that the circulating flu virus will have changed significantly. But this is not usually the case, and even when significant changes occur, the vaccine still offers individuals some protection. That is why WHO strongly recommends its use: "Anywhere between 50% to 80% of vaccine recipients will be protected against the disease when there is a good match between the vaccine and the strains of influenza virus in circulation. Even in those cases when the vaccine does not fully protect against the disease, severity of illness and the frequency of serious complications are reduced."[34]

Methods of Administration

The flu vaccine is administered in two ways—as an injection or as a nasal spray. Injectable flu vaccine consists of dead viruses and is approved for people of all ages. The spray contains

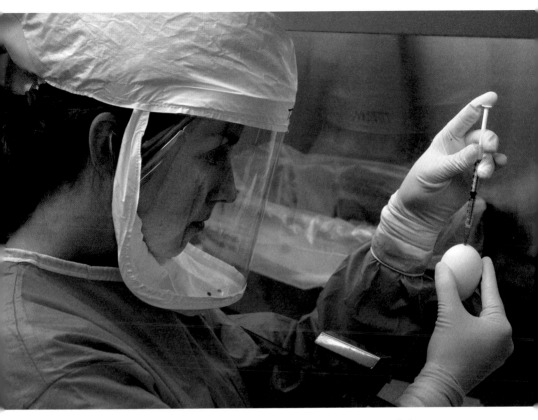

A scientist injects an egg with a mix of viruses as part of the development of a new flu vaccine.

weakened live viruses and therefore presents a risk of infection for people with weakened immune systems, such as individuals with chronic diseases and adults over age forty-five. The spray can also produce asthma-like symptoms in young children and is not administered to children under age five.

Both vaccines are equally effective in preventing the flu. But like all medications, they present some health risks. Pain at the injection site is the most common complaint, and some individuals develop mild flu-like symptoms that last less than twenty-four hours. Complications in the form of allergic reactions can arise for people who are allergic to eggs, because of the way the virus is cultured. These individuals are advised to avoid the vaccine. Some individuals have developed Guillain-Barré syndrome, a serious neurological disorder that causes paralysis, after being administered the flu vaccine. These cases are relatively rare, and scientists do not know what the link is between the condition and the vaccine. Most people, however, think that the benefits of the vaccine far outweigh the risk. One mother, Sheryl, explains:

> Six years ago, my healthy 5 year old son came down with the flu. He hadn't had his vaccine that year. He came desperately close to death and it was the scariest experience in our lives! He is 11 years old now and still remembers his experience with that flu scare and when it comes time every October for his flu shot, he knows that the needle going into his arm could save his life and he is more than happy to get it. . . . I am fortunate that my son survived his near death experience and we were given a second

A four-year-old receives a flu vaccine, which does not prevent all cases of flu but makes getting sick during flu season less likely.

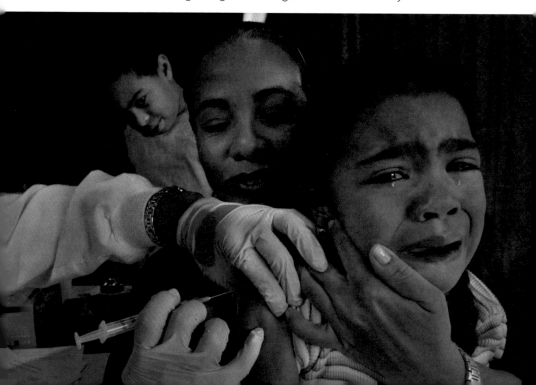

chance. That is why I still today fight tirelessly and with stoic determination to tell all and any parents of healthy children to get their healthy kids vaccinated![35]

Problems with the Vaccine

It takes between two and six weeks for the immune system to respond to the flu vaccine and develop immunity. Therefore, it is best to be vaccinated in October, since the flu season begins in late November in the Northern Hemisphere. Once the immune system responds to the vaccine, if the components of the flu vaccine closely match the circulating flu virus and if the virus does not change radically during the flu season, vaccinated individuals are not likely to develop flu symptoms. If they do, the duration and severity of the infection is usually mild.

However, for a variety of reasons, some people do not choose to be vaccinated. Some individuals avoid vaccination out of worry about possible side effects or because they do not like shots. Others discount the seriousness of the illness, or they doubt they will contract it. Hence, they see no need for protection. Rob is one of these people: "I am strong and healthy, so the flu is not going to kill me. I rarely get sick, so why should I bother getting a shot?"[36]

This makes it difficult for vaccine manufacturers to estimate how many doses of the vaccine will be needed in any given year. Since the vaccine formulation is changed each year, if manufacturers produce more doses of the vaccine than there is demand for, unused vaccine must be discarded. Creating unwanted vaccine can cost pharmaceutical companies thousands of dollars, which is why vaccine manufacturers may not always make enough vaccine to meet the demand. For example, in 2003, 95 million doses of the vaccine were produced for use in the United States, but there was demand for only 83 million doses. The following year, vaccine manufacturers scaled back production. A larger-than-usual flu outbreak in December 2004 caused an unforeseen demand for the vaccine, and shortages occurred. Troubles producing the vaccine compounded the problem.

Due to the possibility of shortages, to ensure that individuals most at risk of developing flu-related complications are protected, the flu vaccine is offered to this group first. Whatever is left is administered to the general public. Although it is not usual, sometimes the demand can exceed the supply. That is what happened to John in 2004 and 2005: "I wanted to get a flu shot the past couple of years but I was unable to. The shots were unavailable in my community for healthy people of my age—under 65."[37]

Social Distancing

Even if vaccine shortages occur, there are still many simple measures unvaccinated individuals can take to guard themselves from infection and infected individuals can take to protect others. These steps provide additional protection for vaccinated persons as well.

Social distancing, a protective measure that simply means avoiding contact with infected people, is one important step. Conversely, infected individuals can protect others by avoiding public places. A single infected student or worker can give the flu to all of his or her peers, who in turn spread it to their friends and families, who spread it in their schools and workplaces, and so on. As a result, it does not take long for one flu case to quickly become one thousand. "When I got the flu, my mom kept me home. I missed school, church, and soccer practice. I couldn't see my friends at school and on the team, but my mom said I was helping others by not spreading my flu germs,"[38] reports one teenager.

Similarly, decreasing contact with items infected people may have touched can also offer protection. Since infectious flu virus particles can linger for days, it is not always possible to identify unsafe items. To be safe, it is best to avoid using public telephones, restrooms, water fountains, and pens provided for customers' use in banks, stores, restaurants, and doctors' offices. Neil Schachter warns: "Each time you go to a

Vitamin C Supplements and Flu Prevention

Many people take high doses of the antioxidant vitamin C in an effort to prevent the flu. The belief that the vitamin prevents infection is based on the work of Linus Pauling (1901–1994), a Nobel Prize–winning biochemist.

According to an article on Wikipedia, in the 1960s, Pauling "began actively promoting vitamin C as a means to greatly improve human health and resistance to disease. His book *How to Live Longer and Feel Better* was a bestseller and advocated taking more than 10,000 milligrams per day."

In the years since Pauling's book, scientific research on Pauling's theory has produced mixed results. Vitamin C does appear to have some antihistamine properties and, like all antioxidants, supports the immune system, but most scientists discount the megadose theory.

The U.S. recommended daily allowance for vitamin C is sixty to ninety milligrams. Citrus fruits such as lemons and oranges contain forty and fifty milligrams, respectively. Other good sources of vitamin C include strawberries, broccoli, kiwifruit, and melons. Since vitamin C is water soluable, large doses are rapidly eliminated from the body, doing little damage. However, excessive dosages can cause diarrhea.

Wikipedia, "Vitamin C." http://en.wikipedia.org/wiki/Vitamin_C.

The late Linus Pauling (pictured here tossing an orange and holding a model of a vitamin C molecule) advocated high doses of vitamin C to prevent flu.

restaurant or store and make a purchase on your credit card, you're offered a pen when you're given your charge receipt. During the flu season, this pen is passed to dozens of people each day and is a superb carrier of . . . viruses. Simply by using your own pen and not lending it out, you can significantly cut down on your exposure to the . . . virus."[39]

Important Health Practices

It is not always possible to avoid contact with infected individuals or potentially contaminated items. But other common-sense health practices can provide protection. Hand washing, for instance, is a good way to protect oneself and stop the spread of infection. People can accumulate flu viruses on their hands through direct contact with infected individuals, through

Vigorous and frequent hand washing is a good way to stop the spread of flu viruses.

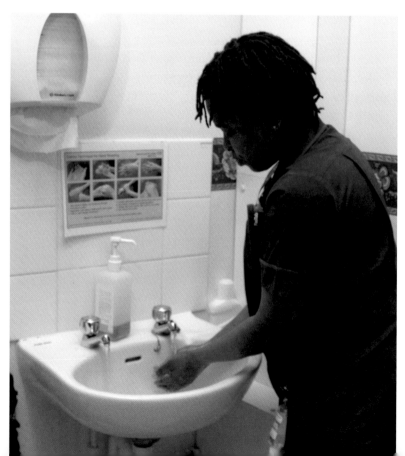

contact with contaminated surfaces, and after sneezing, blowing the nose, or coughing. They can then infect themselves by touching their eyes, nose, or mouth, and they can infect others by direct or indirect contact. To prevent contracting or spreading the flu, medical experts advise people to wash their hands after contact with sick people, sneezing, coughing, blowing their noses, using the bathroom, touching animals and pets, or visiting public places; before eating, drinking, or handling food; and before and after inserting and removing contact lenses. According to many health-care professionals, such behavior is the single best way to prevent the spread of the virus. Yet according to an August 2005 survey conducted by the American Society of Microbiology, only 32 percent of Americans surveyed wash their hands after coughing or sneezing.

Proper hand washing with soap and water loosens viruses on the hands and rinses them away. Medical experts at the Mayo Clinic offer the following instructions:

> Wet your hands with warm, running water and apply liquid or clean bar soap. Lather well. Rub your hands vigorously together for at least 15 seconds. Scrub all surfaces, including the backs of your hands, wrists, between your fingers and under your fingernails. Rinse well. Dry your hands with a clean or disposable towel. Use a towel to turn off the faucet.[40]

In order to know how long to scrub, young children are advised to sing the "Happy Birthday" song, which is about fifteen seconds long.

When soap and water are unavailable, an alcohol-based sanitizer is a good substitute. To be most effective, individuals are advised to apply about one-half teaspoon of the sanitizer to their hands and then rub their hands together until the product dries. If used correctly, alcohol-based sanitizers are as effective as soap and water. That is why this mother carries the product with her: "Keeping my family safe and healthy is my top priority. When we are on the go, running errands or going to a game,

I help protect us from the spread of germs with alcohol-based hand sanitizers to clean hands and faces when we can't get to soap and water."[41]

Coughing, Sneezing, and Touching the Face

Covering the mouth and nose when coughing or sneezing is another practical way to prevent spreading infection. Using the hands to do this is not advisable. Sneezing or coughing into a clean tissue, which should be disposed of immediately, is better. When a tissue is not available, the CDC suggests that people cough into their sleeves. "Coughing into the sleeve of your arm is considered to be safer than coughing into your hands and then spreading the flu that way," explains Marie Kassai. "They're actually recommending that if you're going to wipe your nose, especially for children that they wipe it on their sleeves and not on their hands so that they're not transmitting it."[42]

Keeping the hands away from the mouth, nose, and eyes is another key measure in preventing infection. Since the flu virus can linger on hard surfaces for long periods, people can unknowingly touch infected surfaces, then transport it to the mucous membranes that line these body parts. Phillip T. Hagen, vice chairman of the division of prevention and occupational medicine at the Mayo Clinic, notes: "You often have no choice but to touch things like subway poles and railings. . . . These surfaces are teeming with germs. Scratch your eye without thinking, and you could be setting yourself up [to catch the flu]."[43]

Supporting the Immune System

Another way individuals decrease their risk of infection is by maintaining a healthy lifestyle, which enhances the body's natural defenses. Eating a well-balanced diet rich in fruits, vegetables, legumes, whole grains, and lean proteins is an essential part of this strategy. Fruits and vegetables, in particular, contain a wide variety of essential vitamins and minerals known as antioxidants. These work against damaging substances called free radicals, which attack healthy cells and weaken the immune response.

Drinking at least eight glasses of water a day is also vital. Water plays a significant part in how the body and the immune system function. It aids in the absorption and digestion of food, blood circulation, and the removal of toxins from the body. In addition, without adequate water, the mucous membranes in a person's mouth and throat tend to dry out, making it easier for viruses to attach themselves.

Smoking has a similar effect on the mucous membranes. Moreover, smoking destroys fragile tissues in the lungs and airways, and paralyzes cilia, hairlike substances in the respiratory tract that sweep out viruses and keep them from penetrating the lungs. Smoking also causes mucus to build up in the respiratory tract, providing a perfect breeding ground for the flu virus. And because smoking impairs the ability of white blood cells to fight infection, smokers have weaker defenses than nonsmokers.

As smokers, these teens are more likely to get respiratory infections than nonsmokers.

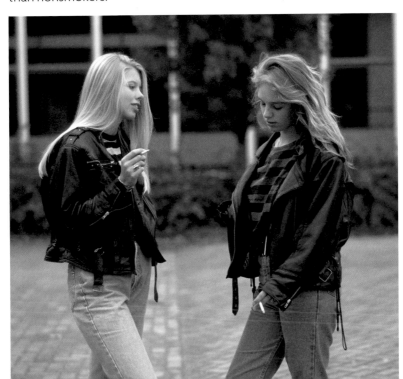

According to health experts at CheckFlu.com, a Web site published by the makers of Tamiflu:

> Smokers are more likely than nonsmokers to get respiratory infections of all types. And when they do get respiratory infections, they often get sicker than nonsmokers do maybe because smoking suppresses immune function. Smoking increases the severity of influenza symptoms and it is recommended that smoking be quit as a preventive measure for influenza.[44]

Indeed, when smokers get the flu, the infection is more likely to penetrate the lungs and cause serious complications and death than in nonsmokers. According to CheckFlu.com, 25 percent of all severe flu-related complications in otherwise healthy adults are linked to smoking. Therefore, another key way to guard against the flu is to avoid smoking.

A county health department employee in Wheaton, Illinois, passes out numbers to people waiting in bitterly cold weather to receive flu vaccinations.

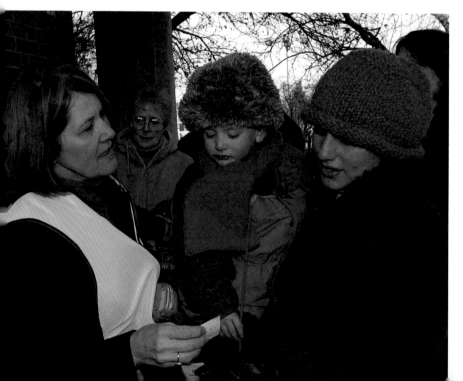

Where to Get a Flu Vaccine

Because public health officials agree that the best way to minimize flu outbreaks is by vaccinating as many people as possible, flu vaccines are administered in numerous convenient locations throughout the United States. In addition to being available in physicians' offices, flu vaccines are administered during scheduled flu clinics for a minimal fee by registered nurses in a wide range of public places. For example, pharmacies and supermarkets often sponsor two or three flu clinics in their stores each season. Frequently, the clinics are scheduled to target peak shopping hours such as in the late afternoon and evening, when working customers can drop in after work. Many businesses, including manufacturers, school districts, hospitals, and large corporations, offer flu vaccines to their employees. These are provided right on the premises, so employees can get vaccinated without taking time out of their busy schedules. When the vaccine is not offered on the premises, some businesses allow workers to leave early so that they can get vaccinated.

Senior citizen centers also offer frequent flu clinics, as do many hospitals. In fact, some hospital flu clinics offer drive-up vaccinations in which nurses vaccinate patients through a car window. In 2005, a drive-up clinic in Oklahoma managed to inoculate nine hundred people in ninety minutes.

Other Strengthening Measures

Getting adequate rest is equally important. Sleep helps the body rejuvenate itself and enables the immune system to function properly. Studies into sleep deprivation show that lack of sleep weakens the immune system and white blood cell production. Consequently, when people are fatigued, they are more vulnerable to infection. Health-care professionals recommend that children and teenagers get nine hours of sleep a night and adults get seven or eight.

Stress, too, weakens the immune system and may increase a person's risk of infection. When people are under stress, production of hormones that interfere with the immune response increases. These hormones decrease the production of white blood cells and inhibit the release of interferon, a protein that hinders viral replication. Developing methods to manage stress helps people counteract its damaging effects. "In peak season for colds and flu," Neil Schachter advises, "try to break the stress buildup by taking time for yourself. Once a day do something that is all about you. Read a magazine or a book, watch a favorite TV show, or meet a friend to help you regroup."[45]

Exercising is a good way to relieve stress. It also boosts a person's immunity. A 2002 study at Iowa State University, for example, found that older adults who get regular and vigorous exercise produce higher levels of anti-influenza antibodies after receiving a flu shot than more sedentary subjects.

Preventive Medicine

Taking preventive medicine is another way individuals protect themselves against the flu. Besides treating flu symptoms, the antiviral medications Tamiflu and Relenza can prevent people who have been exposed to the virus from coming down with influenza. They do this by blocking the spread of the virus in the respiratory tract. A 2005 study conducted by Roche, the manufacturer of Tamiflu, found that the drug provided up to 89 percent protection in adults and teenagers who had been in close contact with flu patients, and 55 percent in children. Once again, because overuse of antiviral drugs may lead to flu viruses developing drug resistance, there is some controversy over their use as a preventive.

It is apparent that there is no way that individuals can completely guard against the flu. But by being vaccinated, practicing commonsense health practices, living a healthy lifestyle, and taking preventive medications, people can reduce their chances of infection. At the same time, infected people can take steps to protect others. In so doing, flu outbreaks can be minimized.

CHAPTER FOUR

Influenza Pandemics

Even when individuals do everything they can to protect themselves from the flu virus, during a flu pandemic it is difficult to control the spread of the disease and prevent infection. Flu pandemics cause high levels of illness and death as well as serious problems for society. The emergence of a new viral subtype, similar to that which caused the worst flu pandemic in history, is a growing concern today.

Unlike seasonal flu outbreaks, which are regional and caused by existing viral subtypes that have changed slightly, pandemics are caused by a new viral subtype that emerges due to antigenic shift. Flu vaccines based on circulating viruses rarely match the new virus, and individuals have little or no antibodies to fight it. Such viruses cause serious infection and spread rapidly throughout the world, causing high levels of illness, death, social problems, and economic loss. CDC epidemiologist Keiji Fukuda explains:

> In terms of infectious diseases, there are very few comparable events to an influenza pandemic. Most infectious diseases have regional or local implications; even a really devastating disease like malaria is confined to warmer areas. There's probably no other disease like influenza that has the potential to infect a huge percentage of the world's population inside the space of a year, and to cause a lot of deaths all over the world.[46]

Crossing the Species Barrier

New viral subtypes that cause flu pandemics form when a human flu virus and a bird, or avian, flu virus exchange, or reassort, their genes and surface proteins. The new virus is unrecognizable to the immune system, which makes it dangerous.

There are more avian flu viruses than there are human flu viruses. Migratory waterfowl such as wild ducks and geese harbor the virus in their intestines, shedding it in their feces. Although the virus may not make these birds ill, it has a devastating effect on domestic poultry such as chickens. According to Rob Webster, the director of WHO's Collaborating Center for Influenza Viruses of Lower Animals and Birds, approximately 30 percent of migrating geese and ducks shed flu viruses in their yearly migration.

Since type A human flu viruses infect other mammals, human and avian viruses can come together inside an intermediary, which is usually a pig. This can happen if a pig roots

Julie Gerberding, director of the Centers for Disease Control and Prevention, attends a national avian flu forum to establish procedures to be used in the event of a U.S. pandemic.

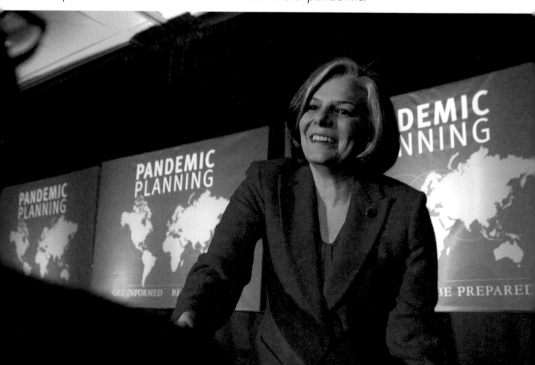

around in contaminated feces. If the pig is also infected with a human flu virus, the two viruses combine. The infected animal then sheds the new virus in its manure, which is transmitted to humans when they come in contact with it. For example, if humans step in contaminated feces, touch their shoes, then touch their eyes, nose, or mouth, the virus gains access to the respiratory tract, causing infection. Some scientists think that the virus that caused the world's most famous flu pandemic in 1918 arose in this manner.

Humans can also acquire the virus directly via contact with contaminated bird feces. If the human is already infected with a flu virus, when the avian virus gains access to the respiratory tract, the two viruses recombine there and a new virus forms.

Like all viruses, the new virus will continue to change over time. Such changes can increase or decrease its virulence. In order to pose a significant threat, the virus must acquire the ability to be transmitted efficiently through human-to-human contact. This can occur when the virus first forms or as the virus changes. Once this happens, the threat of a pandemic arises.

The 1918 Pandemic

There have been ten flu pandemics in the last three hundred years. The 1918 pandemic was the most severe in recorded history. People in every country in the world, with the exception of American Samoa, were infected. In total, one-third of the world's population at that time—about 500 million people—contracted the flu. Between 21 million and 100 million of those infected died, approximately six hundred thousand of whom were Americans. That is more Americans than were killed in all the wars of the twentieth century combined.

No one knows with certainty where the first outbreak of the 1918 flu virus occurred. Although the virus is often called the Spanish Flu because an outbreak in Spain was widely publicized, evidence points to the first outbreak occurring not in Spain but in Camp Funston, Kansas, an army base where soldiers were training for service in World War I. Funston, like all military encampments at the time, was seriously overcrowded, making it a perfect breeding ground for infectious disease. The first cases were reported there on March 4, 1918.

As troops from Camp Funston moved from one jammed army base to another, the virus quickly spread, infecting troops in twenty-four of the largest army camps in the United States and civilians in cities adjacent to the bases. In April, with the arrival of 1.5 million American troops in Europe, the virus spread across that continent. In May alone, more than thirty-six thousand British troops were hospitalized with the illness. A British military report noted: "At the end of May it appeared with great violence. . . . The numbers affected were very great. . . . A brigade of artillery had one-third of its strength taken ill within forty-eight hours, and in the brigade ammunition column only fifteen men were available for duty out of a strength of 145."[47]

It was then carried in trading ships to Australia, Africa, and Asia, where, according to one Chinese witness, "It swept over the country like a tidal wave."[48] Then in June, it returned to the United States. As the virus spread, it became more and more lethal. In the first week of July, it killed 8,287 people in London. In August, it killed 3 percent of the population in the African nation of Sierra Leone. Two months later, in October, it killed 195,000 Americans.

The reason the virus was so virulent was, as it changed, it developed the ability to settle directly in a victim's lungs, hindering breathing and causing severe pneumonia. The body's own inflammatory response damaged the lungs further. Many patients developed blue spots over their face and body because their lungs were so congested that they could not transfer oxygen to their blood. Bleeding from the mucous membranes, which occurred when the immune system attacked blood platelets needed for the blood to clot, was also common. Numerous reports mention patients bleeding profusely from their mouths and noses. Explains author and historian Alfred Crosby:

> One of the factors that made this so particularly frightening was that everybody had a preconception of what the

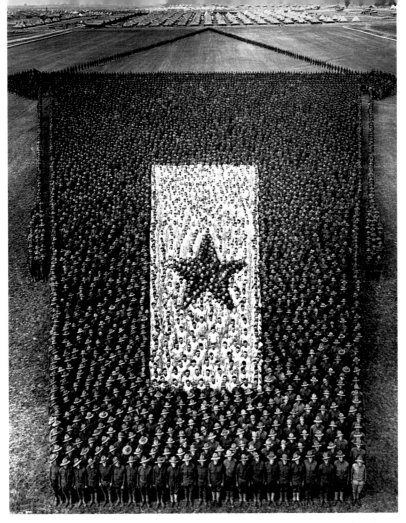

Soldiers stand in banner formation at Camp Funston in 1918. The first flu outbreak of the 1918 pandemic is thought to have started here.

flu was: it's a miserable cold and, after a few days, you're up and around, [but] this was a flu that put people into bed as if they'd been hit with a 2 x 4. That turned into pneumonia, that turned people blue and black and killed them. It was a flu out of some sort of horror story. They never had dreamed that influenza could ever do anything like this to people before.[49]

Because young adults have the strongest immune systems and produce the strongest inflammatory response, this age group was the hardest hit. Their immune response was so extreme that it effectively destroyed their lungs. Indeed, unlike seasonal flu outbreaks where fatalities are greatest in those with the weakest immune systems, in the 1918 pandemic, 40 percent of those who died were between twenty-five and thirty-five years old, an occurrence unique to this particular pandemic. "The situation was upside down and backwards," Crosby notes, "a disease that's supposed to be a mild disease is killing people, the people it's killing are the strongest members, the most robust members of our society."[50]

The Social Impact of the 1918 Pandemic

Besides causing sickness and death, like all pandemics, the 1918 pandemic caused serious social disruption. Because the virus struck so many, there were not enough workers to keep the economy running. As a result, stores, factories, and other businesses were forced to close. This led to shortages of a variety of goods. Daniel Tonkel, who was a child during the pandemic and the son of a storekeeper, recalls: "The first time I was aware that something was amiss in our normal living was when my father told me 'son, most of the employees are sick. We don't have anyone left to run the store. Everyone is home sick or in the hospital sick'. And within a week my father told me that this saleslady had passed away and another one had passed."[51]

Illness also created a scarcity of health-care professionals to tend the sick. To make matters worse, hospitals were overwhelmed. There were not enough medical supplies or beds for all those seeking help, and temporary emergency care centers were set up in parks and town squares. John M. Barry describes the scene at a Massachusetts military hospital: "All the beds had long since been filled. Every corridor, every spare room, every porch was filled, crammed with cots occupied by the sick and dying. . . . And there were no nurses. . . . Seventy out of two hundred nurses were already sick in bed themselves, with more falling ill each hour. Many of them would not recover."[52]

With so many fatalities, wood for coffins and the caskets themselves were in short supply. Coffins became so valuable that funeral homes hired armed guards to protect the boxes from thieves. And because many undertakers were victims of the virus, there were not enough professionals to handle the dead. As a result, in many cities corpses covered with sheets were left out on the street, in gutters, or on front porches for open trucks known as death carts to pick up. The bodies were unceremoniously dumped into large trenches dug by steam shovels that served as mass graves.

Fear of the virus paralyzed cities and towns. People were afraid to leave their homes, and even big cities were like ghost

A shortage of sickbeds for flu victims in 1918 forced the erection of temporary emergency care centers like this tent camp located on hospital grounds.

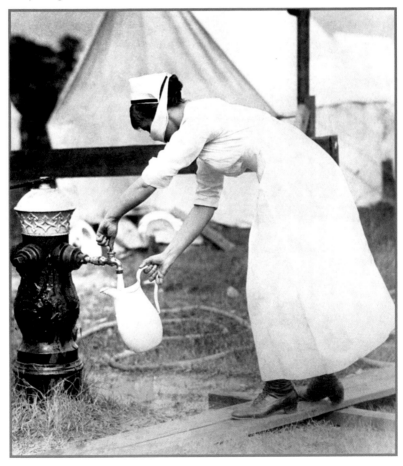

The Pandemic That Never Happened

In February 1976, an eighteen-year-old U.S. army recruit died of the flu. Experts wrongly thought the virus, known as the swine flu virus, was closely related to the virus that caused the 1918 pandemic. In an attempt to deter another pandemic, in October 1976, President Gerald Ford instituted an emergency plan to vaccinate the entire American population against the flu. In order to rush the vaccine to market, the vaccine did not receive as much safety testing as it normally would.

In an article in *Time* magazine, Asia edition, author Bryan Walsh explains what happened: "The inoculation program immediately hit snags. . . . After two months, vaccinations were halted after reports that hundreds of people who had received the shot had developed a rare nerve disease."

Whether the vaccine was at fault was never established. Moreover, there was no actual pandemic threat. The flu death turned out to be an isolated incident.

The article explains: "While the 1976 program was an expensive and embarrassing mistake, it also underscores just how difficult it is to decide how to prepare for an influenza pandemic, whose schedule and severity we have virtually no way of predicting."

Bryan Walsh, "Between Panic and Apathy," *Time*, November 7, 2005. www.time. com/time/asia/news/article/0,9754,1126758,00.html.

towns. Some municipalities instituted quarantines. Schools, churches, theaters, restaurants, bars, and other public meeting places shut down. In an age in which many homes did not have telephones, gathering in these places connected people with each other. As a result, individuals became increasingly isolated. Scientist and infectious-disease expert Laurie Garrett recounts her uncle's experience: "His family insisted that he could not go outside for any reason until the whole epidemic was over. He spent his afternoons looking out the window and counting the hearses going up and down the neighborhood and trying to guess which of his schoolmates had died and keeping a little scorecard."[53]

Orphaned children were reported wandering the streets of some cities, but out of fear of becoming infected, people who would have helped under normal circumstances did not. Indeed, a large but unknown number of children lost one or both of their parents to the illness, and some became homeless.

Even friends and neighbors avoided each other. In some localities, laws were passed requiring people to wear surgical masks, which were poorly constructed and actually offered no protection since the virus could pass through openings in the fabric. Violence erupted against those individuals who ventured out without one. Crosby comments on how a pandemic affects social behavior: "An epidemic erodes social cohesiveness because the source of your danger is your fellow human beings, the source of your danger is your wife, children, parents, and so on. So, if an epidemic goes on long enough, and the bodies start to pile up and nobody digs graves fast enough to put the people into them, the morality starts to break down."[54]

An American police officer dons a facemask in hopes of avoiding flu germs during the 1918 pandemic.

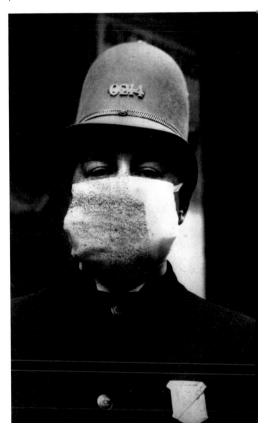

Long-Lasting Effects

Influenza pandemics draw to a close when survivors have developed immunity to the virus and few susceptible victims remain. The 1918 flu pandemic ended in November. The impact of H1N1, the virus that caused the pandemic, however, was not limited to 1918. For the next few decades, slightly changed strains of the virus circulated throughout the world, causing annual flu outbreaks.

In 1957, a descendant of the virus underwent antigenic drift and caused the second flu pandemic of the twentieth century, and a descendant of that virus caused the third pandemic of the twentieth century in 1968. That is why the CDC calls H1N1 the "Mother of All Pandemics."[55]

Neither of these pandemics was as severe as that of 1918. The 1957 pandemic infected approximately 10 to 35 percent of the world's population and killed an estimated 1 to 2 million people worldwide, including about seventy thousand Americans. The 1968 pandemic was the mildest pandemic of the twentieth century. It caused approximately seven hundred

With many students out sick, a nearly empty Dallas, Texas, classroom shows the effects of the 1957 flu pandemic.

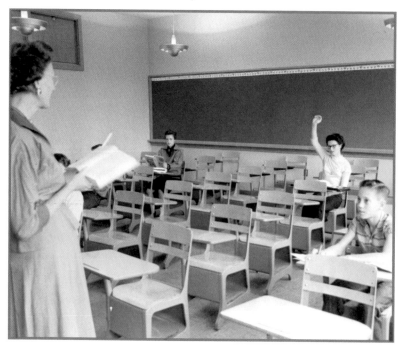

thousand deaths globally, including about thirty-four thousand in the United States. Scientists say that one of the reasons it was relatively minor is that the virus struck in late December during school holidays throughout the world. Consequently, school-age children, who are prime carriers of the virus, did not infect each other at school.

No matter how mild a pandemic, it is still destructive. Hong Kong scientist Paul Saw describes his experience in 1968:

> I went down with it, and it was horrible. It's not the same aches and pains you get with your normal flu, the experience is totally different, I was just knocked out. And I remember, you could see queues [lines] of people at every doctor's office. I think in a three- or four-week period, one-third of the people here were sick. You'd go to the offices, see the vacant desks—and that wasn't a very serious one. A really major one . . . I wouldn't even dare to think.[56]

Scientists do not know for certain why the 1957 and 1968 pandemics were less catastrophic than the 1918 pandemic. Scientific analysis of each virus's genes has shown some interesting differences, which scientists theorize affected the way victims reacted to the different pathogens. The 1918 virus was largely a bird virus that upon reassortment incorporated the capacity to infect humans and spread via human-to-human contact. To put it simply, much like a child who closely resembles one parent, H1N1 closely resembled its avian parent. This made H1N1 totally unfamiliar to the human immune system. The later viruses, on the other hand, were mainly human viruses that took on some avian characteristics, making them less unfamiliar and hence less dangerous.

The Avian Flu

In 1997, H5N1, another avian flu virus, emerged. It is like H1N1 in that it is unrecognizable to the human immune system; but it differs in one significant way—as of March 2006, H5N1 could only cause infection in humans through contact with sick birds. Nevertheless, scientists and public health officials quickly became concerned about the possibility that it could acquire the capacity to be spread person-to-person, sparking a pandemic.

The H5N1 virus first appeared in Hong Kong, killing thousands of chickens. Shortly thereafter, eighteen people became infected and six died. In an effort to thwart a pandemic, the Hong Kong government ordered the culling, or slaughter, of all poultry in the nation. One and a half million animals were destroyed. No other infections were reported, and it seemed like a public health disaster was averted until the virus reemerged in 2003, carried by migratory wild birds.

By March 2006, it had virtually exploded, infecting chickens, ducks, turkeys, and swans in Asia, Africa, the Middle East, and Europe, with more countries reporting cases almost daily. Commenting on the devastating spread, WHO spokeswoman Maria Cheng says: "We've never seen so many outbreaks of the same virus in so many different regions. Our concern obviously is that humans could potentially come into contact with birds infected with H5N1, which would mean populations worldwide are potentially at risk."[57]

As the virus spread, it became more pathogenic, killing bird species that are normally not receptive to the viral strain. Over 200 million birds died or have been destroyed as a result of the illness, causing huge economic losses in the form of lost jobs and revenue. For example, in 2004, the bird flu cost Asia over $10 billion. And because chicken is an important food in Africa, where the virus was first detected in 2006, these losses are expected to skyrocket and cause serious food shortages across the continent. The United Nations (UN) Food and Agricultural Organization chief veterinary officer, Joseph Domenech, describes the extent of the problem: "This highly pathogenic avian influenza virus poses a very serious threat to animal health in West Africa. If a poultry epidemic should develop beyond the boundaries of Nigeria [the first African country to be infected] the effects would be disastrous for the livelihoods and food security of millions of people."[58]

How Deadly Is the Bird Flu?

Although the bird flu appears to have killed more than 50 percent of its human victims, a January 2006 study at Karolinska University Hospital in Stockholm, Sweden, suggests that the virus is more widespread and less harmful than experts think. But because many cases are relatively mild, the cases are not reported.

The study involved 45,476 residents of a rural region of Vietnam where the bird flu is widespread in poultry. Eighty percent of the subjects lived in households that kept poultry, and one-quarter reported sick or dead birds in their flocks.

According to an Associated Press article,

A total of 8,149 reported flu-like illness with a fever and cough, and residents who had direct contact with dead or sick poultry were 73 percent more likely to have experienced those symptoms than residents without direct contact.... While most patients said their symptoms had kept them out of work or school, the illnesses were mostly mild, lasting about three days.

Although this study is encouraging, because blood samples were not taken to confirm that the subjects were indeed infected with bird flu, the results are not conclusive.

Associated Press, "Research: Bird Flu More Common, Less Deadly," *Las Cruces Sun News*, January 10, 2006, p. 3A.

In this same period, at least 177 human cases have been reported, and these numbers appear to be rising sharply. Indeed, in less than two weeks in January 2006, 16 human cases were reported in Turkey alone, in comparison to 143 cases worldwide before that time. As with the 1918 virus, H5N1 penetrates deep into victims' lungs, and those most susceptible are otherwise healthy children and young adults. As of March 2006, there have been 98 deaths. This translates to a 55 percent fatality rate, the most lethal of any influenza outbreak ever.

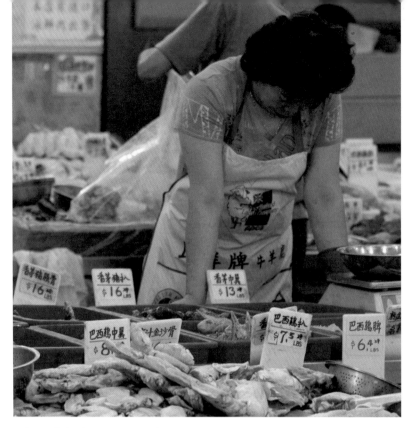

Sales of chicken are slow for this vendor in Hong Kong, where the avian flu virus first appeared.

As bad as this may be, health officials worry about the threat of the virus developing the capacity to be passed easily between humans. If that should happen, another pandemic, with the potential to be even more lethal than that of 1918, is likely to arise. Laurie Garrett notes: "What's scaring us is that this constellation of H number 5 and N number 1, to our knowledge, has never in history been seen in our species. So absolutely nobody watching this has any natural immunity to this form of the flu."[59]

Scientists cannot predict whether the virus will change enough for this to occur. But it is clear that any time an avian flu virus exchanges surface proteins with a human flu virus, acquiring the capacity to infect humans and spread easily, a pandemic occurs. Illness, death, and global societal problems follow.

CHAPTER FIVE

Preparing for the Next Flu Pandemic

Based on the nature of the influenza virus and historical precedent, health experts say that it is not a matter of *if* another flu pandemic will occur in the future, but rather *when*. "This is not a probability issue," explains Michael Osterholm, the director of the Center for Infectious Disease Research and Policy at the University of Minnesota, Minneapolis. "It's going to happen. What we don't know is which strain it's going to be or when it's going to happen. It could be tonight. It could be ten years from now."[60]

A twenty-first-century pandemic is likely to begin in Asia, where humans often live in close contact with domesticated and wild animal populations. Such an event may have more devastating consequences than the 1918 pandemic. Even if the percent of infection and mortality rates is the same, based on the current world population, an estimated 180 million to 360 million people could die, including 1.7 million Americans. And according to the Lowry Institute, an Australian think tank, global economic losses could top $4.4 trillion.

Governments, health organizations, and scientists throughout the world are working together to respond to such a threat in an effort to minimize the damage it could cause. "People have to understand that this is not science fiction," Osterholm warns. "Pandemics are going to happen. This is why a group of

infectious disease experts are trying to wake the world up. . . .
The bottom line is we have a lot to do to get better prepared."[61]

The Avian Flu Threat

Many experts expect that the H5N1 virus will cause the first flu
pandemic of the twenty-first century. According to scientists,
H5N1 is continually adapting. Such changes can lessen the
virus's potential to do harm or enhance its power. One significant change has expanded the range of animals the virus in-

The next flu pandemic could start in Asia, where people like this
Vietnamese woman live in close proximity to birds and other
animals.

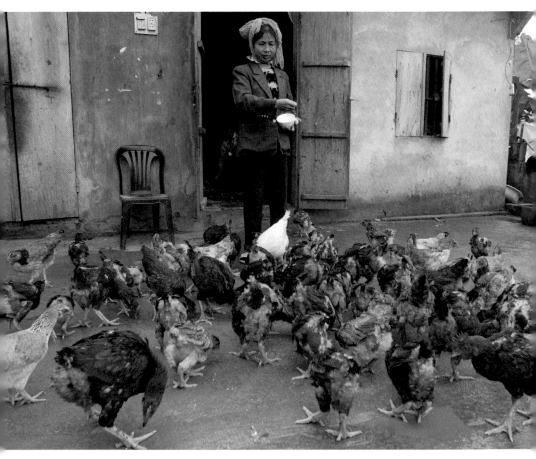

fects. Robert Webster, an influenza researcher at St. Jude Children's Research Hospital in Memphis, Tennessee, says that H5N1 "is probably the worst influenza virus, in terms of being highly pathogenic, that I've ever seen or worked with. Not only is it frighteningly lethal to chickens, which can die within hours of exposure, swollen and hemorrhaging [bleeding profusely], but it kills mammals from lab mice to tigers with similar efficiency."[62] In fact, the virus killed over one hundred tigers in Thailand in 2005. It has also been detected in cats and dogs.

Tests by WHO scientists in Turkey in January 2006 disclosed that other changes in the virus allow it to attach to and penetrate human cells more easily than in the past. "It's a little concerning because the virus is still trying new things in its evolution,"[63] notes Michael Perdue, director of WHO's response team.

Because H5N1 is so changeable, scientists theorize that it may develop the ability to be transmitted readily from person to person on its own. David Nabarro, UN coordinator for avian and human influenza, notes: "There are some subtle changes in the genetic makeup of H5N1 which suggest that it is making some of the mutations that would enable it to have a higher likelihood of being able to become a human-to-human transmitted virus."[64]

Moreover, with the virus spreading rapidly throughout the world, more animals and humans are coming in contact with it. The more contact, the more likely that H5N1 will get into the respiratory tract of a pig or human infected with a human flu virus and acquire the transmissibility trait it currently lacks. "We cannot tell when the mutation might happen, or where it might happen, or how unpleasant the mutant virus will turn out to be," Narbarro explains. "Nevertheless, we must remain on high alert for the possibility of sustained human-to-human virus transmission and of a pandemic starting at any time."[65]

Spreading with Unprecedented Speed

Whether the avian flu virus or another influenza virus is responsible for the next flu pandemic, experts warn that modern patterns of transportation and demographic changes mean it is likely to spread more rapidly and cause more damage than any previous pandemic.

International air travel, today more rapid and generally more affordable, can spread an influenza virus at a rate that was never before possible. An estimated half a billion people board planes each year in the United States alone. If there is an outbreak of a dangerous influenza virus anywhere in the world, an infected passenger can carry it across international borders in a matter of hours.

In 1918, it took six to nine months for H1N1 to circle the globe. According to WHO, a modern pandemic with human-to-human transmission could spread to every continent in less than three months and could find its way to most major cities in one to three weeks. The time factor is important, because in such a scenario an influenza virus would have little chance to weaken naturally over time. Because people are crowded into airplanes, where the air is constantly recirculating, commercial air flights provide an ideal breeding ground for influenza. Just one infected individual could easily infect everyone on a flight, each of whom could pass the virus on.

Making matters worse, since people are contagious before developing symptoms, unless large-scale quarantines prohibiting all air travel are instituted, efforts to keep infected people from flying would be largely ineffective. Explains Bill Karesh, the lead veterinarian for the Wildlife Conservation Society: "It's going to come out of Bangkok or Hanoi or Hong Kong or Shanghai, get into Japan. It'll get to New York. It'll get to San Francisco. It'll get to Vancouver. It'll get to Paris and London, all within a matter of the first week."[66]

Another key factor is the rise in world population. It was 1.8 billion in 1918; today it exceeds 6 billion, therefore representing a vastly larger pool of potentially susceptible victims. Not only that, more people live in crowded urban areas than ever before, making it easier for infectious diseases to spread. Forty-three percent of the world's inhabitants live in cities with a population of at least five hundred thousand.

Many of these cities are in developing nations, where poverty, malnutrition, limited sanitation, and inadequate medical care are a way of life. According to WHO, one-third of the world's population lacks access to essential health care, and an estimated one out of every three children in developing nations suffers from malnutrition, which weakens their ability to resist epidemic diseases.

Ongoing wars and social unrest add to the problem. Famine and strife throughout the world has displaced millions of people, forcing them to live in unsanitary, overcrowded resettlement

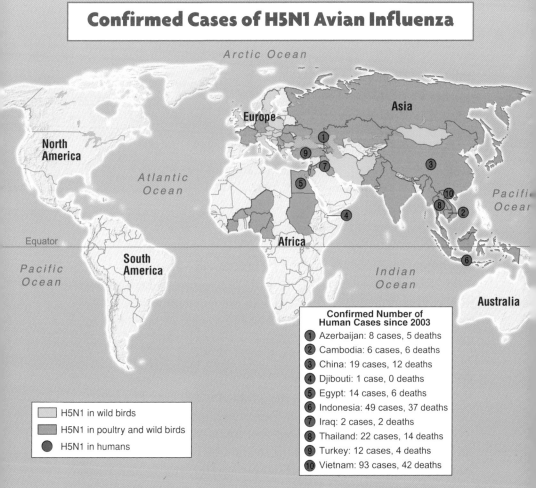

Confirmed Cases of H5N1 Avian Influenza

Confirmed Number of Human Cases since 2003

1. Azerbaijan: 8 cases, 5 deaths
2. Cambodia: 6 cases, 6 deaths
3. China: 19 cases, 12 deaths
4. Djibouti: 1 case, 0 deaths
5. Egypt: 14 cases, 6 deaths
6. Indonesia: 49 cases, 37 deaths
7. Iraq: 2 cases, 2 deaths
8. Thailand: 22 cases, 14 deaths
9. Turkey: 12 cases, 4 deaths
10. Vietnam: 93 cases, 42 deaths

H5N1 in wild birds
H5N1 in poultry and wild birds
H5N1 in humans

Sources: U.S. Department of Health & Human Services (www.pandemicflu.gov) and World Health Organization (www.who.int). Data from 2003 through May 2006.

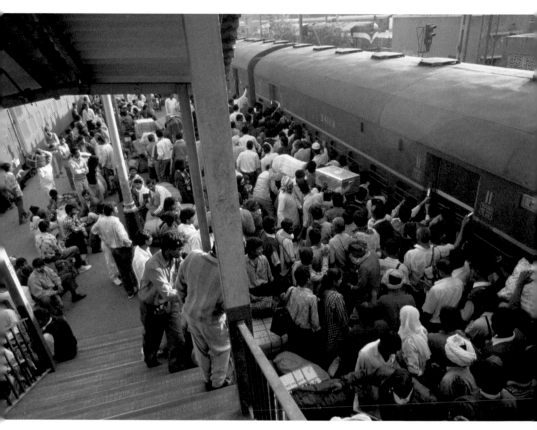

Infectious diseases spread more easily in crowded cities such as New Delhi, India (pictured).

and refugee camps, where poverty and disease are rampant. At least two of these camps in Sudan house more than eighty thousand people each. These people are especially vulnerable to infection, and their movement can help spread influenza to new areas.

Social Consequences

Not only is a twenty-first-century pandemic expected to infect more people than ever before, the social consequences are potentially more devastating. Demand for medical services will far exceed the supply. According to John M. Barry, "Even in advanced countries a pandemic would stretch the health care system to the point of collapse. . . . In developing countries the health care system would all but disintegrate."[67]

As many as 10 million Americans are likely to need hospital care, but due to budgetary constraints, the United States has fewer hospital beds per person than it did during the 1968 pandemic. Life-support equipment is also in short supply. Currently, there are 105,000 mechanical ventilators in the United States, all of which are utilized during normal seasonal flu outbreaks. Many more will be needed in a pandemic.

Drugs and other medical supplies may also be limited. International, national, and local quarantines are predicted. Since one of the best ways to prevent infection is minimizing contact with others, quarantines are part of the U.S. Department of Health and Human Services (HHS) Pandemic Influenza Plan, released in November 2005. As a result, air and sea cargo shipments are likely to be curtailed. Because an estimated 80 percent of all drugs use raw materials from foreign sources, essential medications may be delayed or unable to reach their destination.

What is more, due to the fact that modern businesses function on what is known as a just-in-time supply chain, in which supplies are ordered as needed rather than stockpiled, a disruption of global trade will upset supply chains, and entire industries will be crippled. This will lead to scarcities of a multitude of other products ranging from computer chips to food. Because most modern people depend on food being brought in from external sources, severe food shortages are predicted. Moreover, since most cities purify their water with chlorine, if shipments of that chemical are delayed, shortages of drinking water could occur. That is why government officials are advising Americans to store at least a week's worth of nonperishable food, water, and medical supplies.

Quarantines will also mean the closing of schools and mass transit. Isaac Weisfuse, New York City's deputy health commissioner, notes: "People talk about 'flu days' like snow days and if it was just days or weeks, that would be simple. But if it's weeks or months, that becomes another matter. Without mass transit, no one gets to work and the economy collapses. And many poor children depend on the free breakfasts and lunches they get at school."[68]

Reducing the Threat

Governments, health organizations, and scientists throughout the world are taking a number of steps to respond to the threat of a pandemic. Some of the steps are specific to the avian flu, while others are more general. These steps should minimize the damage such an event could cause.

WHO is taking the lead in these actions. In addition to analyzing circulating viral samples in order to determine the components of a vaccine, its Global Influenza Surveillance Network

A World Health Organization official speaks at a press briefing following a 2005 avian flu conference in Ho Chi Minh City in Vietnam.

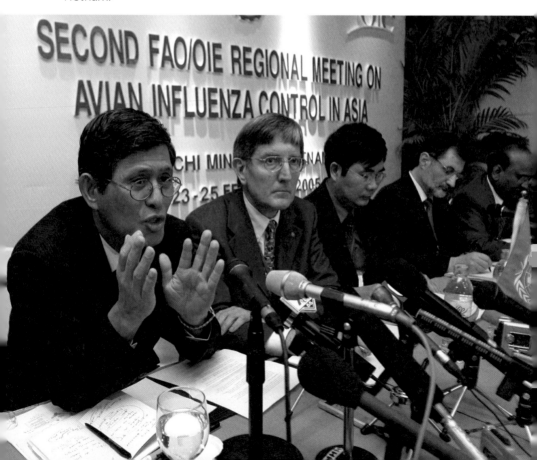

Detecting Bird Flu in Humans

At the present time, blood tests, which involve analyzing blood samples in a laboratory, are the only way to establish the presence of a particular flu virus in an animal or human. Such tests can take two to three days. But scientists are developing a number of new ways to detect the presence of H5N1 rapidly in humans. This would enable health agencies to identify the source of infection and begin control and prevention activities more rapidly, which would help contain a pandemic.

One novel method created by STMicroelectronics, a Paris company, uses a microchip that can establish the presence of bird flu within an hour. The chip functions much like a dipstick. A blood sample or a swabbing taken from inside an individual's nose or throat is placed on the chip. It is then read by a machine programmed to identify H5N1.

Tests have shown the process to be 99 percent accurate. The manufacturer hopes to market the apparatus to airports and immigration points, where sick people will be quarantined. This would help keep infected people from spreading H5N1 across international boundaries. The device could also be used in hospitals as a rapid diagnostic tool. It should be available in late 2007.

acts as a mechanism for identifying new viruses. Network scientists track flu outbreaks, gather blood samples from infected individuals, and analyze viral characteristics. If a new viral strain is detected, epidemiologists from WHO's Global Outbreak Alert and Response Network (GOARN), whose job it is to investigate the transmission and control of epidemic diseases, interview victims and medical personnel in order to learn more about the virus. For example, in an ongoing investigation, GOARN scientists are gathering blood samples of residents of Turkish villages infected with avian flu. By analyzing the samples, they hope to establish whether people are carrying the virus or show antibodies to it. This will help them learn

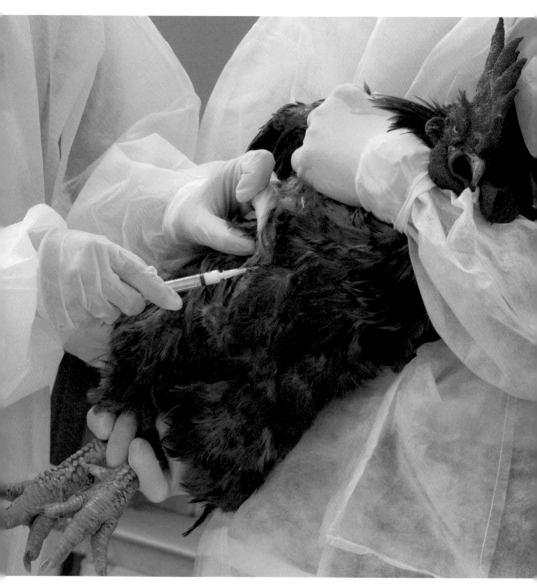

Chinese health authorities vaccinate a domestic chicken against bird flu.

more about how the virus is spread and develop and fine-tune strategies aimed at controlling it. In addition, GOARN team members ensure that appropriate technical assistance is provided to infection sites so that containment measures can be implemented. The CDC, which focuses on the United States, assists WHO and performs a similar function in America.

Containing Outbreaks

One important strategy aims to minimize human infection by containing outbreaks of H5N1 in poultry and wild birds. This is being done in a number of ways. First, migrating waterfowl are being monitored. For example, U.S. spy satellites are tracking infected flocks. And animal influenza experts at the U.S. Department of Agriculture (USDA) maintain surveillance of migratory birds in western Alaska that share breeding grounds with Asian birds. Since 1998, the scientists have analyzed twelve thousand wild bird fecal samples for the presence of H5N1 in North America. Project scientist David Swayne notes: "Over eight years, we have not found any H5N1 viruses. That's good news."[69]

The USDA plans even more aggressive surveillance and testing in 2006. The scientists are planning to test between seventy-five thousand and one hundred thousand live and dead birds as well as five times more fecal samples than it has screened since 1998. And the testing zone will be extended to include some Pacific islands. "We'll have to keep vigilant,"[70] Swayne explains.

Domestic birds are also being watched closely. In countries where H5N1 has been detected, poultry flocks in which an infected bird has been found have been destroyed. Some nations have destroyed all domestic flocks in a certain radius of an infected area as a precaution. For instance, 800,000 birds in western India, 455,000 birds in twenty-six Turkish provinces, and 11 million birds in parts of Thailand were killed following local outbreaks. "We're trying to break the link between birds and humans by destroying fowl,"[71] explains Hurrem Bordur, a Turkish health official.

Other measures are also in effect. Many countries have quarantined infected areas in order to control the movement of infected birds. Vehicular inspections aimed at keeping contaminated birds from being transported out of an affected region are part of this plan. To be extra cautious, vehicles leaving infected regions in France must first pass through a long trough, where they are disinfected. At the same time, infected farms throughout the world have been treated with disinfectants. And many nations have tightened border controls and surveillance. The European Union, for example, banned the importation of live or dead poultry from infected nations, as did Japan.

Keeping poultry indoors and vaccinating domestic flocks are other ways to contain the virus. Millions of birds have already been vaccinated in Vietnam and Thailand. In 2005, China instituted an ongoing program to vaccinate 5.2 billion chickens, geese, and ducks in that nation, while the European Union approved a poultry vaccine plan for member nations in February 2006.

Indeed, world leaders consider containing H5N1 so critical that nations throughout the world have pledged $1.9 billion to the World Bank. That organization will distribute the money to needy countries to help cover the costs of mass culling, compensation to farmers, and animal vaccinations.

Changing Human Behavior

Changing risky behaviors is another key strategy. In many parts of the world, people live in close proximity to domestic poultry. Children often play with backyard flocks and come in close contact with bird feces. In cold weather, the animals may be brought inside the house. Many domestic flocks are not kept penned in and are allowed to roam freely. This increases their chances of coming in contact with infected wild birds and spreading the virus. Worse still, due to poverty, sick birds are not always discarded but killed, plucked, and eaten instead. Contact with an infected animal's blood can spread the virus.

Many people in developing nations are unaware how dangerous these behaviors are. Therefore, federal governments and health professionals from a wide array of organizations are working together through media campaigns as well as door-to-door visits in an effort to educate people in ways to reduce behaviors that can lead to infection. Speaking in Nigeria, United Nations Children's Fund spokeswoman Christine Jaulmes cautions: "It is only an improvement in healthy behaviours among families and communities that could prevent a transfer of the bird flu to humans, especially children."[72]

Improving Preparedness

At the same time, governments, health organizations, and scientists throughout the world are taking steps to minimize the damage a pandemic may cause by improving preparedness. Indeed, most nations and every state in the United States have

In many developing nations, people like this Asian boy feeding his family's chickens are often unaware of behaviors that may lead to bird flu infection.

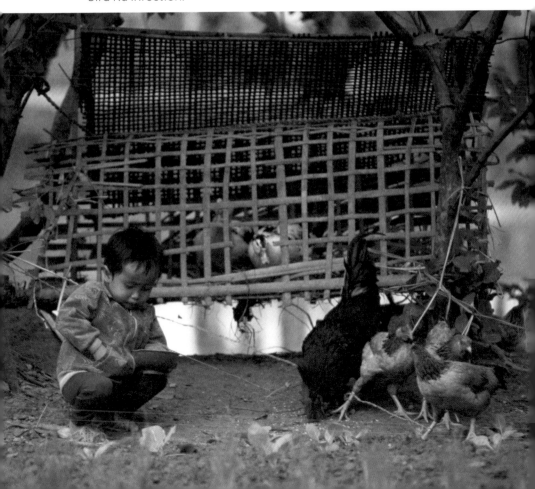

Flu Vaccines Should Get to Market Sooner

Because of the long time it takes for a flu vaccine to be developed and approved for distribution, the U.S. Food and Drug Administration (FDA), which regulates all drugs in the United States, has proposed new guidelines that will speed flu vaccines to market. The guidelines promote research into new, faster-growing vaccines, encourage vaccine manufacturers to develop and store vaccines against multiple flu strains in an effort to have vaccines available against new viral strains, and allow for rapid emergency approval of new vaccines should a pandemic arise.

The guidelines allow manufacturers to modify already-approved flu vaccines for use against a new flu subtype without having to regain FDA approval, which was required in the past. In addition, according to an article on CNN.com, "a manufacturer could receive accelerated approval for a new flu vaccine by performing studies that showed that the recipients experienced a surge in protective immune-system cells." In the past, recipients were tracked to see if they caught the flu before approval was granted, which was a much slower process.

According to the head of the FDA's vaccine office, the agency's goal is to "make sure we have the capacity to make enough influenza vaccine . . . for everyone who needs it."

CNN.com, "FDA to Speed New Flu Vaccine to Market," March 3, 2006. www.cnn.com/2006/HEALTH/conditions/03/03/birdflu.fda.ap/omdex.html.

pandemic preparedness plans. And many localities, including New York City and Seattle, have run influenza-specific drills simulating mock outbreaks in an effort to increase emergency preparedness. They then used the results of the drills to improve their plans.

Developing new preventive medications and treatments as well as improving access to antiviral drugs are important elements of preparedness plans. For example, in March 2006,

WHO had a global stockpile of 2.5 million treatment courses of Tamiflu. By May 2006, that number is expected to rise to 3 million. Similarly, the United States is adding to its supply and hopes to acquire enough antiviral drugs to treat 75 million Americans. Sixty-five other countries have placed similar orders to fill their pandemic stocks. Explains U.S. secretary of Health and Human Services Michael O. Leavitt: "Having a stockpile of antiviral drugs is an important part of our pandemic influenza preparedness plan."[73]

A special face mask, which can filter out 95 percent of all viruses, is also being stockpiled in the United States, and in the event of a pandemic outbreak in the country, localities are likely to pass regulations requiring their use in public areas. More efficient than surgical masks, these masks would be distributed to the public to help prevent the virus from spreading.

At the same time, research scientists are working on developing new drugs. One group at the biotechnology company NexBio in San Diego is investigating a type of drug known as a fusion protein. It works by fusing to receptor cells in the respiratory tract, thereby blocking all flu viruses from attaching to the cells and gaining access to the airways. The drug, which is called Fludase, is administered as an inhalant. So far, animal tests have been quite promising, and human trials are scheduled to begin in 2006. If Fludase proves to be effective, because it is not specific to a particular flu virus, it will be a valuable weapon in combating new viral strains.

Developing a Vaccine

Pharmaceutical companies are working on developing a vaccine that protects humans against H5N1. Indeed, two trials of two separate bird flu vaccines were set to begin in the spring of 2006. If the vaccines prove to be effective, they should be available by 2008.

At the same time, a novel vaccine is currently being developed at the University of Pittsburgh. Rather than being cultured in fertilized eggs, which takes up to six months to complete, this vaccine is made by using laboratory-grown bird flu proteins and takes only thirty-six days to develop. It is then placed into a genetically modified, harmless cold virus and injected into the body. So far, animal studies have shown it to be 100 percent effective in preventing infection.

Interestingly, the vaccine not only stimulates the creation of antibodies but also activates the production of virus-fighting white blood cells. As a result, even if the targeted virus changes radically, the vaccine offers more protection than traditional vaccines that must match circulating viruses. Study

Turkeys await evaluation in Israel. In March 2006 Israeli officials confirmed that thousands of turkeys and chickens on two farms had died of avian flu.

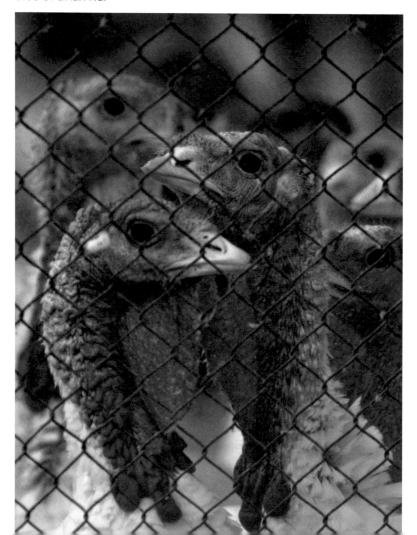

codirector Andrea Gambotto explains: "Using this technology we can have much broader protection, which is important because the virus is always changing."[74]

Although experts warn that another flu pandemic is inevitable, governments, scientists, and health organizations throughout the world are working together to respond to the threat. "What we have to do for pandemic flu preparedness is better prepare our world to get the living through it, the sick through it, and then come out the other end as well as we possibly can. That's the difference between hopelessness and hopefulness,"[75] warns Michael Osterholm.

Preparations like the development of new vaccines and antiviral medications, the stockpiling of drugs, flu outbreak surveillance, the creation of preparedness plans, and the culling, vaccination, and monitoring of animals provide hope that even if a flu pandemic strikes, its severity will be minimized. "We're learning things everyday," explains John Stephens, New Hampshire's Health and Human Services commissioner. "We cannot be satisfied until our plans are the best they possibly can be to protect the public health."[76]

Notes

Introduction: An Underrated Problem

1. Quoted in Pete Davies, *The Devil's Flu*. New York: Henry Holt, 2000, p. 63.
2. Neil Schachter, *The Good Doctor's Guide to Colds and Flu*. New York: HarperCollins, 2005, p. 153.
3. Marilyn, telephone interview with the author, Brooklyn, NY, February 6, 2006.

Chapter 1: What Is Influenza?

4. Davies, *The Devil's Flu*, p. 75.
5. Schachter, *The Good Doctor's Guide to Colds and Flu*, p. 23.
6. John C. Brown, "The Flu is a Bummer." http://people.ku.edu/~jbrown/flu.html.
7. John M. Barry, *The Great Influenza*. London: Penguin, 2005, p. 110.
8. Barry, *The Great Influenza*, p. 110.
9. Quoted in ABC News, "Good Behavior During Flu Season." http://abcnews.healthology.com/webcast_transcript.asp?b=ab/1cnews&f=infectiousdiseases&c=infect_flu prevent&spg=SCH.
10. John, personal interview with the author, Las Cruces, NM, February 10, 2006.
11. Marilyn, telephone interview.
12. Quoted in MSNBC.com, "ERs Are Packed as Flu Outbreak Hits Arizona," December 28, 2005. www.msnbc.msn.com/id/10624216.
13. Marilyn, telephone interview.
14. Quoted in Families Fighting Flu, "Connecting with Others." www.familiesfightingflu.org/connect/view.aspx.
15. Quoted in NBC10.com, "Flu Shots for Pregnant Women."

www.nbc10.com/health/2701554/detail.html.

16. Quoted in ABC News, "Cold and Flu Smarts." http://de
troitnews.healthology.com/webcast_transcript.asp?b=
detroitnews&f=children&c=children_flukids&spg=SCH.

Chapter 2: Flu Symptoms, Diagnosis, and Treatment

17. Sammy, telephone interview with the author, Mount
Kisco, NY, February 12, 2006.

18. Liam, telephone interview with the author, Mount Kisco,
NY, February 12, 2006.

19. Liam, telephone interview.

20. Sammy, telephone interview.

21. Sammy, telephone interview.

22. Rob Hicks, "Flu (Influenza)," BBC. www.bbc.co.uk/
health/conditions/flu1.shtml.

23. Schachter, *The Good Doctor's Guide to Colds and Flu*,
p. 158.

24. Joan Morris, "Get Some Rest," *Albuquerque Journal*, January 16, 2006, p. C1.

25. Schachter, *The Good Doctor's Guide to Colds and Flu*,
p. 48.

26. Liam, telephone interview.

27. Liam, telephone interview.

28. Quoted in CBC News, "Is Chicken Soup Good Medicine?"
January 16, 2001. www.cbc.ca/consumers/market/files/
food/chickensoup.

29. Quoted in World Famous Recipes, "Chicken Soup
Recipes." www.worldfamousrecipes.com/chicken-soup-
recipes.html.

30. Quoted in MSN.com, "Home Humidifiers: Soothe Your
Nose, Throat, and Skin." http://health.msn.com/guides/
coldandflu/articlepage.aspz?cp-documentid=100096401.

31. Schachter, *The Good Doctor's Guide to Colds and Flu*,
p. 50.

32. John, personal interview.

Chapter 3: Preventing Influenza

33. Quoted in Amanda Gardner, "Universal Flu Shots Urged," MSN Health and Fitness. http://healthmsn.com/guides/coldandflu/articlepage.aspx?cp-documentid=100110421.
34. WHO, "Recipe for the Northern Hemisphere Flu Vaccine," February 16, 2000. www.who.int/inf-pr-2000/en/pr2000-08.html.
35. Quoted in Families Fighting Flu, "Connecting with Others."
36. Rob, personal interview with the author, Las Cruces, NM, February 21, 2006.
37. John, personal interview.
38. Quoted in CDC, "Real People." www.cdc.gov/flu/toolkit/stories/flubreak.htm.
39. Schachter, *The Good Doctor's Guide to Colds and Flu*, p. 70.
40. Mayo Clinic, "Hand Washing: A Simple Way to Prevent Infection." www.mayoclinic.com/health/hand-washing/HQ00407.
41. Quoted in CDC, "Real People."
42. Quoted in ABC News, "Good Behavior During Flu Season."
43. Quoted in Kristyn Kusek, "No More Colds or Flu," *Good Housekeeping*, January 2002. http://magazines.ivillage.com/goodhousekeeping/hb/health/articles/0,,284594_408716,00.html.
44. CheckFlu.com, "Smoking and Influenza." www.checkflu.com/smoking_and_influenza.html.
45. Schachter, *The Good Doctor's Guide to Colds and Flu*, p. 229.

Chapter 4: Influenza Pandemics

46. Quoted in Davies, *The Devil's Flu*, p. 17.
47. Quoted in Barry, *The Great Influenza*, p. 170.
48. Quoted in Barry, *The Great Influenza*, p. 172.
49. Quoted in PBS, *The American Experience:* "Influenza 1918." Program Transcripts, p. 5. www.pbs.org/wgbh/

amex/influenza/filmmore/transcript/transcript1.html.

50. Quoted in PBS, *The American Experience*, p. 15.

51. Quoted in PBS, *The American Experience*, p. 6.

52. Barry, *The Great Influenza*, p. 189.

53. Quoted in *Primetime*, "Are We Ready for the Bird Flu?" ABC News, September 29, 2005. http://abcnews.go.com /Primetime/Flu/story?id=1170177&page=2.

54. Quoted in PBS, *The American Experience*, p. 18.

55. Jeffrey K. Taubenberger and David M. Morens, "Emerging Infectious Diseases," CDC. www.cdc.gov/ncidod/eid/vol 12no01/05-0979.htm.

56. Quoted in Davies, *The Devil's Flu*, p. 38.

57. Quoted in *Las Cruces Sun News*, "International Health Experts Concern over Bird Flu Spread," February 22, 2006, p. 10A.

58. Quoted in Steven R. Hurst, "Egypt Confirms Bird Flu as Virus Spreads," *Albuquerque Journal*, February 18, 2006, p. A9.

59. Quoted in *Primetime*, "Are We Ready for the Bird Flu?"

Chapter 5: Preparing for the Next Flu Pandemic

60. Quoted in *The Oprah Winfrey Show*, "The Next Pandemic?" Oprah.com, January 24, 2006. www.oprah.com/to ws/slide/200601/20060124/slide_20060124_284_101.jhtml.

61. Quoted in *The Oprah Winfrey Show*, "The Next Pandemic?"

62. Quoted in Tim Appenzeller, "Tracking the Next Killer Flu," National Geographic.com, October 2005. www7. nationalgeographic.com/ngm/0510/feature1.

63. Quoted in *Albuquerque Journal*, "Bird Flu May Pose Bigger Risk," January 12, 2006, p. A6.

64. Quoted in Flu Wikie, "Expert Opinions About a Flu Pandemic." www.fluwikie.com/index.php?n=Science.Opinion AboutAFluPandemic.

65. Quoted in *Las Cruces Sun News*, "Bird Flu Virus Spreads in Nigeria, Azerbaijan," February 11, 2006, p. 12A.

66. Quoted in *Primetime*, "Are We Ready for the Bird Flu?"

67. Barry, *The Great Influenza*, p. 453.

68. Quoted in Donald G. McNeil Jr., "Greetings Kill: Primer for a Pandemic," *New York Times*, February 12, 2006. www.nytimes.com/2006/02/12/weekinreview/12mcne.html ?ex=1141534800&en=d02. . . .

69. Quoted in Amy Cox, "Scientists Look to Other Species for Some Human Flu Answers," CNN.com, November 14, 2005. www.cnn.com/2005/HEALTH/11/14/flu.animals/ index.html.

70. Quoted in Cox, "Scientists Look to Other Species for Some Human Flu Answers."

71. Quoted in William Kole, "WHO Wants to Do Massive Flu Survey in Turkey," *Albuquerque Journal*, January 14, 2006, p. A7.

72. Quoted in Crofsblogs, "UNICEF Advises Nigerian Parents," March 4, 2006. http://crofsblogs.typepad.com/h5n1.

73. Quoted in Gardiner Harris, "U.S. Stockpiles Antiviral Drugs, but Democrats Critical of the Pace," *New York Times*, March 2, 2006. www.nytimes.com/2006/03/02/poli tics/02flu.html?_r=1&oref=alogin.

74. Quoted in Jennifer Bails, "Bird Flu Breakthrough," PittsburghLive, January 27, 2006. www.pittsburghlive.com/x/ tribune-review/trib.pmupdate/s_417589.html.

75. Quoted in *The Oprah Winfrey Show*, "The Next Pandemic?"

76. Quoted in ABC News, "New Hampshire Gets Ready for Bird Flu." www.abc.news.go.com/GMA/FLU/story?id= 1331258.

Glossary

antibody: A naturally occurring protein produced by the immune system to defend the body from foreign substances.

antigen: A substance that activates the production of an antibody when it enters the body.

antigenic drift: Small changes in the surface proteins of a virus.

antigenic shift: Abrupt and major changes in the surface proteins of a virus.

antiviral medications: Drugs that inhibit viruses from attacking the body.

avian flu (bird flu): An infectious form of influenza that normally affects only birds.

culling: The selective killing of animals to protect the herd or species.

cytokines: Proteins that initiate an inflammatory response that produces fever and body aches.

epidemic: A local, regional, or national disease outbreak.

hemagglutinin: One of two proteins that surround the RNA core of the flu virus.

histamines: Inflammatory substances that cause congestion, sneezing, and coughing.

H1N1: The virus that caused the 1918 flu pandemic.

H5N1: The avian flu virus that is currently circulating.

inflammation: The body's response to infection. It is characterized by heat, redness, and swelling and often elicits the symptoms of influenza.

neuraminidase: One of two proteins that surround the RNA core of the flu virus.

pandemic: A worldwide disease outbreak.

ribonucleic acid (RNA): The genetic material that forms the core of the flu virus.

social distancing: Avoiding contact with infected individuals as well as avoiding public gatherings.

vaccine: A medication that creates immunity to particular illnesses by exposing the immune system to a small dose of greatly weakened or inactivated (dead) pathogens.

virus: A microscopic parasite that invades the body and causes disease.

white blood cells: Cells whose job it is to attack and destroy foreign substances in the bloodstream.

Organizations to Contact

American Lung Association

61 Broadway, 6th Fl.
New York, NY 10006
(800) LUNG-USA
Web site: www.lungusa.org

The association provides information about all respiratory diseases, including the flu.

Centers for Disease Control and Prevention (CDC)

1600 Clifton Rd. NE
Atlanta, GA 30333
(800) CDC-INFO
e-mail: cdcinfo@cdc.gov
Web site: www.cdc.gov/flu

The influenza branch of the CDC provides a wealth of information on the flu, including fact sheets, information on how the virus spreads, vaccines, flu prevention, outbreaks, pandemic awareness, and avian flu. It also works to control and track flu outbreaks.

Immunization Action Coalition

1573 Selby Ave., Suite 234
St. Paul, MN 55104
(651) 647-9009
e-mail: admin@immunize.org
Web site: www.immunize.org

This organization works at ensuring that people are vaccinated for a wide variety of illnesses. It has a number of good flu-related links on its Web site.

National Foundation for Infectious Diseases

4733 Bethesda Ave., Suite 750
Bethesda, MD 20814
(301) 656-0003
e-mail: info@nfid.org
Web site: www.nfid.org

This organization works to prevent infectious diseases. It offers information about what the flu is, how it is diagnosed and treated, prevention, and vaccinations.

National Institute of Allergy and Infectious Diseases

6610 Rockledge Dr., MSC 6612
Bethesda, MD 20892
(301) 496-5717
Web site: www.niaid.nih.gov

This Web site offers information about various infectious diseases, including influenza.

World Health Organization (WHO)

Avenue Appia CH-1211
Geneva 27, Switzerland
011-41-22-791-2111
e-mail: infor@who.ch
Web site: www.who.int/topics/influenza/en

The main agency of the United Nations concerned with global health problems, WHO tracks flu outbreaks through its FluNet, compiles and releases statistics and research reports, helps national public health agencies develop pandemic plans, and offers a wealth of information about avian flu to the general public.

For Further Reading

Books

Virginia Aronson, *The Influenza Pandemic of 1918*. Langhorne, PA: Chelsea House, 2000. An informative young adult book dealing with the 1918 pandemic.

Donald Emmeluth, *Influenza*. Langhorne, PA: Chelsea House, 2003. Talks about the influenza virus and flu epidemics.

Jeffrey N. Sfakianos, *Avian Flu*. Langhorne, PA: Chelsea House, 2006. A look at the avian flu.

Alvin Silverstein, Virginia B. Silverstein, and Laura Silverstein Nunn, *The Flu and Pneumonia Update*. Berkeley Heights, NJ: Enslow, 2006. Discusses the causes, treatment, and prevention of pneumonia and flu.

Lisa Yount, *Epidemics*. San Diego: Lucent, 2000. Looks at the causes and consequences of epidemics, with a section on influenza pandemics.

Periodicals

Tim Appenzeller, "Tracking the Next Killer Flu," *National Geographic*, October 2005.

Christina Gorman, "How Scared Should You Be?" *Time*, October 17, 2005.

Kristyn Kusek, "No More Colds or Flu," *Good Housekeeping*, January 2002.

Anthony Spaeth, "Revenge of the Birds," *Time*, February 9, 2004.

Internet Sources

The Oprah Winfrey Show, "The Next Pandemic?" Oprah.com, January 24, 2006. www.oprah.com/tows/slide/200601/200601 24/slide_20060124_284_101.jhtml.

PBS, *The American Experience:* "Influenza 1918." www.pbs.

org/wgbh/amex/influenza/filmmore/transcript/transcript1.
html.

Web Sites

ABCNews (www.abcnews.go.com/Health/Flu). Dozens of articles about seasonal and avian flu, interactive videos, statistics, and flu-related television show transcripts.

Flu Wikie (www.fluwikie.com). A Web site dedicated to influenza, with a wide array of links to articles, current events,
news archives, statistics, pandemic preparedness information, and expert opinions.

FluWire (www.fluwire.com). Collects news articles from
around the world on the avian flu.

**International Information Programs, U.S. Department of
State** (http://usinfo.state.gov/gi/global_issues/bird_flu.ht
ml). Articles on bird flu and what steps the United States is
taking to prepare for and respond to a pandemic, including
the HHS Pandemic Influenza Plan.

MSNBC (msnbc.msn.co/id/4067116). The Web site has a large
section on the avian flu, including the latest news, interactive videos, slide shows, and time lines.

Index

Picture Credits

Cover photo: Chris Bjornberg /Photo Researchers, Inc.
Maury Aaseng, 20
© allOver photography/Alamy, 34
AP/Wide World Photos, 46, 86
© Bettmann/CORBIS, 66
© Derek Brown/Alamy, 70
© CORBIS, 61
© Creasource/CORBIS, 11
Andrew Davies/Photo Researchers, Inc., 14 (image)
Deep Light Productions/Photo Researchers, Inc., 40
© Jonathan Ernst/Reuters/CORBIS, 58
© foodfolio/Alamy, 38
James Gathany/CDC, 43
© Alex Hofford/epa/CORBIS, 80
© Jeremy Horner/CORBIS, 76
© Jose Luis Pelaez, Inc./CORBIS, 24, 33
Greg Knobloch/CDC, 45
© Adrees Latif/Reuters/CORBIS, 78
© Robert Maass/CORBIS, 83
© Tannen Maury/EPA/epa/CORBIS, 54
© Mika/zefa/Corbis, 9
Hoang Dinh Nam/AFP/Getty Images,72
Susumu Nishinaga/Photo Researchers, Inc., 18
Pasieka/Science Photo Library/Photo Researchers, Inc., 17
Photos.com, 23, 30
© Picture Partners/Alamy, 53
© plainpicture GmbH & Co. KG/Alamy, 29
© Roger Ressmeyer/CORBIS, 49
© Syner-Comm/Alamy, 50
Topical Press Agency/Hulton Archive/Getty Images, 65
© Underwood & Underwood/CORBIS, 63
© Allana Wesley White/CORBIS, 27

About the Author

Barbara Sheen has been an author and educator for more than thirty years. She has written more than twenty-five nonfiction books for children and young adults. Her work has been published in the United States and Europe. She lives in New Mexico with her family. In her spare time, she likes to swim, garden, and cook.

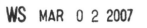